CW00505880

This book is for you if...

- you are searching for some inspiration in your day-to-day life

- you are looking for an educational yet fun read on happiness

- you need practical advice and exercises to help you find your inner happiness

- you want to immerse yourself in a journey of discovery that will help you find your true self

- you are hoping for a thought-provoking read

- you crave motivation to galvanise you into action

- you want an interactive guide that you can dip in and out of at your leisure

- you want to delve into a book that takes you on a journey with help, support and love

- you need to explore some new recipes and motivational moves to get you fitter and healthier

- you wish to learn some life-changing tools that will help you connect with your mind, body and soul

- you need help to find a fresh start to living a happier life

"In her book, *Live Happy*, Rebecca Myers presents an all-inclusive description of what it means to be happy in the modern age. She demonstrates this with a comprehensive story of the neurobiological, social and emotional influences on happiness. Alone, this is impressive, but to do it in such an accessible and engaging way is inspiring! Rebecca peppers her absorbing text with examples from her life, others' lives and quotations from thought leaders, to produce a well-rounded description of the foundations of happiness. Finally, there are numerous practical (and fun!) exercises for the reader to take part in. Even just reading the book puts a smile on your face!"

Dr Eoin Harty
Consultant Anaesthetist
North West London Hospital

"*Live Happy* is an inspiring, educational and practical book. Rebecca Myers has managed to combine scientific fact with a more light-hearted view of happiness, including some heartfelt and honest examples of her own. *Live Happy* is a thoroughly enjoyable read! It not only provides interesting insight into – let's face it – what we are all trying to aim for in our lives, but delivers the information in a bite-sized and manageable way, keeping the reader engaged throughout.

Well done, Rebecca! Can't wait to see what you follow this up with next!"

Isabella Mevola
Regulatory Strategy Director
Pfizer UK

"What an amazing book! Rebecca Myers explores the meaning of happiness, including many personal experiences that engage the reader and help them to explore their own journey, with an understanding that they are not alone! It's wonderful to be able to pick up a book that covers these topics and not feel preached to but instead find help and support, or a simple reminder, whilst taking one's own personal journey. I love *Live Happy*!"

Brook Nolson
Chief Operating Officer
Inspiration Healthcare Group Plc

"Practical, inspiring, and uplifting, *Live Happy* connects the history of happiness research and turns it into practical life-changing tools that allow us to connect with our mind, body and soul. This level of self-awareness is life-altering with a network of deep human connection and support. Rebecca Myers has been my personal trainer and coach, and has helped me create healthier and happier workplaces. Most importantly, she is one of my deep human connections. Live Happy!"

Sarah Kleinpeter
Vice President
Novo Nordisk

"In *Live Happy*, Rebecca Myers invites the reader to embrace the idea that we all deserve the opportunity to be happy, and that we have the capacity to make that happen. Neatly balancing philosophy and theory with real-life examples and practical advice, Rebecca has distilled and blended ideas and perspectives from an eclectic mix of sources, as well as her own experience in the corporate world and as a personal trainer and wellness entrepreneur. There is something for everyone in this book from nutritious recipes and endorphin-boosting movement, to happiness cultivating exercises; all fuelled by Rebecca's own infectious energy and enthusiasm."

Antonia Boyce
Director, In-House Counsel
Leading Global Media Company

"*Live Happy* embodies a positive can-do attitude. It is a clear manual offering a wide variety of tools from which to choose; aimed at making you feel happier by making your body feel great.

Rebecca Myers has been my personal trainer for two years. I did not aim to become an 'ultra-endurance athlete' but I did aim to get fitter, and I am on that road, getting a little further every day. The added benefits I pick up on my road to fitness are those great 'happiness chemicals' which never fail to improve my mood and make me smile. I attribute this to a mix of exercise, great advice from Rebecca, and positive delivery."

Julie Hutchison
Global Asset Lead
Ipsen Bioinnovation Ltd

"Upon receipt of Rebecca Myer's book, *Live Happy*, I was more than a little intrigued by its holistic 'triangular' approach to life's journey. The book is well-researched, factual and data-rich, yet it maintains a freshness and not-too-serious tone, resulting in an enjoyable and fulfilling read. Get on the triangle wherever it suits and start wherever it feels right. Joining the dots of Feel, Move and Eat has been a real pleasure and I'm now looking forward to putting *Live Happy* into practice."

Phil Wharam
Managing Director of Vineuse Ltd,
Author of award-winning novels and screenplays: 'Greed', 'Right to Live', and 'Mengele'

"In this guide, Rebecca Myers effortlessly transitions between delving into the science behind our own happiness, to practical tips on how to spark happiness in the day-to-day. As someone who can't live without a to-do list (!), I especially loved the round-ups of each chapter with advice and steps to take to translate some of these learnings into real life. I flew through the book, finding myself nodding along to the questions Rebecca poses to her readers. Do we know happiness without suffering? How important is resilience in our quest for happiness? What should I cook for dinner?! While I don't claim to have all the answers yet, *Live Happy* has given me a kick-start to my own version of sustainable happiness – in a way that works for me! Thank you, Rebecca, for this Ultimate Guide!"

Mary Ellen
Senior Manager, Operational Strategy,
Multinational Technology Company

"I have known Rebecca Myers for over 14 years, and she has always been a source of incredible energy; able to successfully juggle a family life, as well as being an entrepreneurial businesswomen. *Live Happy* is a valuable resource for anyone seeking to enhance their well-being and provide a catalyst for the action they need to embark on their journey to a happier life. It is truly the pinnacle of who Rebecca truly is. I believe that when one door of happiness closes, we often look so longingly at the closed door, that we do not see the new door that has just opened. This book brings that to the forefront... So, dive in, learn something new, and embrace all that makes you personally happy. Enjoy the journey, and live happy!"

Perminder Gray
Founder and Creative Director
Another Level Medispa
(Bringing Inner and Outer Wellness of Mind, Body, Spirit and Soul)

"*Live Happy* brilliantly dissects the concept of happiness, offering practical advice and thought-provoking insights. From finding joy in simple moments, to exploring the impact of work and relationships on our well-being, Rebecca Myers' book is a valuable guide to living a fulfilling life. It's a must-read for anyone seeking to balance the triangle of life and discover the true essence of happiness. Highly recommended!"

Susan Howard
Psychiatric Nurse and Holistic & Aesthetic Practitioner

"*Live Happy* explores the concept of finding and keeping happiness. It delves into the science of happiness, the external factors that contribute to our joy, and the actionable steps we can take to find and sustain those positive emotions. You can either read it cover to cover for a deep understanding, or pick it up whenever you need a dose of inspiration and guidance. Rebecca Myers is passionate about her work, and her commitment to helping us find happiness shines through every page. She takes a down-to-earth and practical approach, providing readers with tangible advice to enhance their daily lives. Whether you are looking for dinner inspiration, a new workout routine, or a deeper understanding of life, *Live Happy* has you covered. Whether you take away one positive message or adopt several life-changing habits, this book is a valuable addition to your reading list."

Gemma Leeks
University Lecturer

Your Ultimate Guide To Becoming a
Happier Human

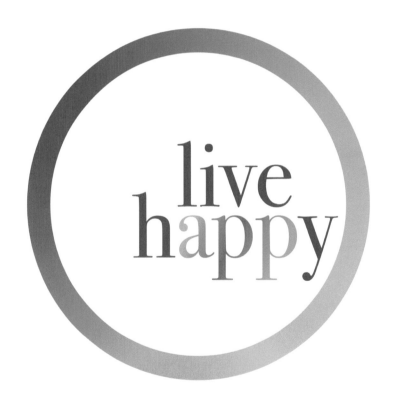

live
happy

Rebecca Myers

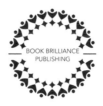

First published in Great Britain in 2023
by Book Brilliance Publishing
265A Fir Tree Road, Epsom, Surrey, KT17 3LF
+44 (0)20 8641 5090
www.bookbrilliancepublishing.com
admin@bookbrilliancepublishing.com

© Copyright Rebecca Myers 2023

The moral right of Rebecca Myers to be identified as
the author of this work has been asserted in accordance with
the Copyright, Designs and Patents Acts 1988.

All rights reserved. No part of this publication may be
reproduced, stored in a retrieval system, or transmitted, in any
form or by any means without the prior written permission of the
publisher, nor be otherwise circulated in any form of binding or
cover than that in which it is published and without similar condition
being imposed on the subsequent purchaser.

A CIP catalogue record for this book is available
at the British Library.

ISBN 978-1-913770-78-5
Printed by 4edge Ltd

This book is not intended as a substitute for the medical advice
of physicians. The reader should regularly consult a physician in
matters relating to his/her health and particularly with respect to any
symptoms that may require diagnosis or medical attention.

To Sam. For putting up with me for 20 years.

To Mum, Dad and Caroline. For putting up with me for 40 years.

CONTENTS

FOREWORD

*L*ive Happy is a feeling that we all want to experience in our lives. This book uniquely illustrates how we can do that when we choose to take action to create lasting change. Rebecca Myers uses her training, experience and expertise to find a fun and lasting way to embrace happiness.

When you ask 'why' you should do something, finding evidence that clearly illustrates that answer is essential. In *Live Happy*, Rebecca expresses the reasons, benefits and lasting change that takes place when you decide to do something different. As she demonstrates, it's about commitment to being your best version and finding a path that quickly leads you to Live Happily with consistent action. Finding that *joie de vivre* that Rebecca enjoys is contagious, as she takes the reader on a passionate and compelling journey.

The book's cleverly crafted structure engages the reader with ease, and the advice is precise and clear on how they can connect to their happiness. With three main themes – Feel, Move and Eat – each individual chapter finishes with a call to action for the reader to engage in. *Live Happy* is not simply a book offering advice. It embraces a multi-media, multi-sensory approach with a QR code taking the reader directly to Rebecca as she demonstrates how to do all of the exercises included on the pages of the Move section.

I believe including the recipes is an innovative approach to everything Rebecca discusses and shares within the book. As these are her recipes, they have certainly been tried and tested and look delicious! The recipes can also be found on Rebecca's Live Happy app.

It is clear to see and feel that Rebecca is passionate about her work, which is more than a career; it is her purpose, and she gives the very best of herself based on her own experiences. She has not just shared her story but provides other evidence of why she believes in what she teaches. This transparent approach will leave the reader with no doubt that Rebecca is an authentic expert in her chosen field of fitness and well-being.

Packed with personal anecdotes and examples, *Live Happy* is a book that will take the reader on a journey of truth and discovery.

Roderick Martin
Co-owner and CEO of GO2 Health, Australia

Rod is dedicated to the health and well-being of others. He founded GO2 Health, arguably the most dynamic and broad-ranging health space in Australia. GO2 integrates many different types of care to ensure the most effective treatment for patients, including general practice, nursing, psychiatry, physiotherapy, acupuncture, massage, psychology, dietetics and exercise physiology. He is also an acupuncture practitioner, a member of the Chinese Medicine Board of Australia, and has degrees in Microbiology, Health Science and Business. Rod has risen to 7th Dan Gojuryu Seiwakai and JKF Japan karateka and is a Hoshindo karate chief instructor.

www.go2health.com.au

INTRODUCTION

Why do we strive to do what we do? Why do we prefer to do certain activities more than others? Why do we prefer spending time with some people (or pets) than others? Why do our bodies react in certain ways depending on what we do or eat? Why, why why!! These are some of the questions I get asked all the time. I believe it all boils down to finding and keeping happiness.

"The pursuit of happiness: More success, more money, more friends – all to come closer to our goal in life: happiness. But once we have it, we are still not always satisfied. We want to experience this feeling again and again, even if it might become too much of a good thing. We are not satisfied with the condition of satisfaction... Happiness is rather a state of continuous pursuit." (The Happiness Project)

YOU are the reason I am very happy in my job – my wonderful clients (past and present), my social media followers, my gym members, the people who have attended my webinars and conferences, and last but not least, YOU, my readers. You have made the effort to interact with me, and I am much happier and better for it. This book is for you, dear reader! If you take away one positive and helpful message, I will have done my job! So, take your time to read this book, learn something new, and try to do as many things as you can that make you personally happy!

I haven't gone too deep or spiritual – I didn't want to write an academic or an ethereal book! For example, if you want some inspiration for dinner, then turn to the Eat section. If you are bored in the gym and want a new workout suggestion, then flick to the Move section. However, if you are struggling to understand life a bit at the moment and want further depth and explanation, start at the beginning and work your way through. At the end of each chapter is a summary as well as mini exercises (Action Time) to practise what you have read. Look out for the little Rebecca avatar!

> *"Action may not always bring happiness,*
> *but there is no happiness without action."*
> Benjamin Disraeli (1804 – 1881)
> British Prime Minister and writer

When thinking about happiness, my first port of call was to turn to facts and science. I realised that I needed to conduct a survey. I surveyed over 100 people of different demographics, gender and age, and asked them the simple question,

"What makes you happy?"

The results were as follows:

- Spending time with family and friends

- Walking in nature (countryside, mountains, beach)

- Pets (in particular dogs)

- Exercising/looking after their health

- Hobbies

- Seeing other people happy (particularly their children)

- Food (either eating out or certain foods such as chocolate)

- Addictions (cigarettes, alcohol)

- Spending time on their own

- Listening to music

- Holidays/travelling

- Achieving goals/winning (small and large)

I wasn't particularly surprised about any of the answers, but was pleasantly surprised about how quickly people responded – they were very pleased to discuss this topic and it made them feel proud to say so.

How to use this book:

Section 1, Feel, is dedicated to delving into the above answers in much more detail – why do these, in particular, come top of our list and what can we change to do more of it? I also look at the opposites; what makes us unhappy – I have called this anti-happiness.

Section 2, Move, delves into further detail about what makes our bodies feel better, with some gym and home-based exercise ideas for you to try as well.

Section 3, Eat, features some yummy and healthy recipes for you to experiment with, and talks about different food groups and how to eat better for a happier life.

Enjoy and live happy!

Rebecca

FEEL

1 A – DEFINING HAPPINESS

What is 'happiness'?

Let's start with a bit of science. What, from a scientific perspective, is happiness? Happiness is a state of mind that has been described in many ways. To pick a few of my favourite definitions:

The Oxford English Dictionary definition is simply: *"the state of feeling or showing pleasure, or the state of being satisfied that something is good or right."*

In her book *The How of Happiness*, Sonja Lyubomirsky, a noted positive psychology researcher, used a definition that I also liked, that goes into a little more depth: *"Happiness can be defined as an enduring state of mind consisting not only of feelings of joy, contentment, and other positive emotions, but also of a sense that one's life is meaningful and valued."* (Lyubomirsky, 2007)

Kendra Cherry, MSEd, defines happiness in an article she wrote for the Verywell Mind website: *"Happiness is an emotional state characterized by feelings of joy, satisfaction, contentment, and fulfilment."*

In all of these definitions, there is an overlap. Happiness is a feeling that we strive to attain. This section is called Feel for a reason and goes into a level of detail as to why we want these feelings and what we do to continue getting them.

Happiness and research

The great philosopher and polymath Aristotle was probably the first to study happiness in great detail. A pupil of Plato and founder of the first scientific institute, the Lyceum, based in Greece, Aristotle's teachings regarding the science of happiness were the most advanced of their time. One of his most influential works is the *Nicomachean Ethics*. In these lectures, he sought to answer "What is the ultimate purpose of human existence?" That is to say, what is the end goal for which we should direct our activities? Aristotle would argue that happiness is the end goal of every person, and after my research, study and experience of the human interactions and goals I have witnessed, I would certainly agree with him 2,300 years later!

"Happiness is the meaning and purpose of life, the whole aim and end of human existence."

Aristotle (384 BC – 322 BC)
Greek philosopher and polymath

He suggested four levels of happiness:

Level 1 – happiness from material objects

Level 2 – ego happiness, from comparison and doing better or being more admired by others

Level 3 – happiness from doing good for others

Level 4 – perfect happiness

The last level is hard to describe but could be considered as finding a spiritual connection to the larger universe.

Some believe that happiness is a result of our circumstances, while others argue that it is entirely within our control. However, in recent years, the science of happiness has emerged as a field of study that provides a more detailed understanding.

Although Aristotle may have started the science of happiness, the advancements in this area of study are vast. Studies have found that happy people are less prone to sickness and stress, and have a better overall well-being. There are many examples of this, but the following story in a paper by Steven Greer & Maggie Watson truly highlights the reason why. The paper suggests that being happy and having a positive attitude could help heal.

"A 24-year-old happily married woman who complained of a mole which had enlarged and begun to bleed was diagnosed as having a malignant melanoma. She was found to have metastasis disease. She was started on intensive cytotoxic therapy but responded only partially. She insisted on knowing her likely prognosis. When she was told she had two years at the most, she declared, 'I will prove them to be wrong,' and she said she would continue to live a normal life. This she did to the great surprise of the clinicians involved in her care. She is still alive and well four years later. She is convinced that her (positive) attitude has pulled her through, since other patients who were diagnosed at the same time as having malignant melanoma or an equivalent stage, have already died." (Greer & Watson, 1987)

Research has also identified several factors that contribute to our happiness, including positive relationships with others and remaining social. From 1938, the comprehensive and groundbreaking happiness study of Adult Development by Harvard University has been gathering health records and detailed interviews about the lives of 724 participants. The latest report concluded: *"The most consistent finding we've earned through 85 years of study is: Positive relationships keep us happier, healthier and help us live longer."*

One of the key factors is our social connections. People who have a strong social support network tend to be happier and live longer lives. Vibeke Koushede, Professor and Head of the Department of Psychology University of Copenhagen, states:

"Ultimately, the good life is about something as simple as having someone or something to get up for in the morning. This is true whether we are young or old. We simply need each other." (Happiness Research Institute, 2002)

Additionally, factors such as financial stability, good health, and satisfying work contribute to long-term happiness. I discuss each of these in more detail in later chapters.

Are you aware of what is happening in your body to make you feel happy? It's all about wonderful and very clever chemicals!

Happiness chemicals

When we experience happiness, our bodies release a variety of natural chemicals that contribute to our overall sense of well-being. One of the primary chemicals involved is dopamine. Often referred to as the 'feel-good' neurotransmitter, dopamine plays a crucial role in reward and pleasure systems in the brain. It is responsible for the sense of motivation, pleasure, and reinforcement we feel when something positive or rewarding happens in our lives. Dopamine also helps regulate our mood, memory, and attention, leaving us with a sense of happiness and contentment. Smelling your favourite perfume, watching your child's face when they accomplish a task for the first time, or hearing your absolute favourite song playing on the radio – all of these things instantly release dopamine!

Another chemical released during moments of happiness is serotonin. Serotonin is a neurotransmitter that influences our mood, appetite and sleep, among other functions. It is often referred to as the 'happiness hormone' due to its role in promoting feelings of well-being and contentment. Balanced serotonin levels contribute to a stabilised mood and a sense of calmness, allowing us to experience happiness and emotional stability.

Furthermore, endorphins, known as 'feel-good' neurotransmitters, are also released during moments of happiness. Endorphins act as natural painkillers and stimulate feelings of pleasure and euphoria. They are responsible for the 'runner's high' experienced during intense physical exercise and contribute to a sense of well-being and relaxation. If you are at the gym and have completed a great run or weights session, you may be hot and sweaty and your muscles may feel tired, but you have a strong feeling of satisfaction, pleasure and positivity. That's your endorphin chemicals kicking in! It happens time and time again as well, so means that you want to keep going. We are clever, aren't we?

These chemicals work in combination to create the sensation of happiness, promoting positive emotions, motivation, and overall well-being. They help reinforce positive behaviours, encourage social bonding, and contribute to the overall balance of our mental and emotional state. Watch out, they are addictive!

This is a quote from one of my clients after she finished her first Sprint Triathlon and the happiness chemicals were flowing strongly:

"This sense of achievement is overwhelming! If you had asked me six months ago if I would ever be able to complete a triathlon, I would have laughed in your face. But I have done it. I've DONE IT!!! You believed in me and I am so happy!"

But will my client feel the same way if she completes a second and third triathlon? Do the chemicals work the same way when we repeat something we find extreme happiness in? The concept of hedonic adaption would perhaps suggest they wouldn't.

Understanding hedonic adaptation

I believe the concept of hedonic adaptation is crucial to understanding our happiness levels. Hedonic adaptation is a psychological phenomenon when our brain gets used to the changes in our environment, and the effects of positive events fade away over time. For instance, getting a new job or buying a new car can bring happiness initially, but the effects will soon dwindle away.

Hedonic adaptation is based on the idea that humans have a natural tendency to adapt to their circumstances, whether positive or negative, and that their initial response diminishes over time as they become accustomed to these circumstances. This adaptation process has been observed across various life domains, including relationships, wealth, material possessions, and even life-altering events.

For instance, imagine winning a significant amount of money or purchasing a material possession that you have long desired – that new car you have had your eye on for ages! Initially, this change may bring an immense amount of pleasure and happiness. However, over time, you might notice that the level of happiness or satisfaction you get from that money or possession diminishes, and you return to your baseline level of well-being. Similarly, if you were to experience a negative event, such as a job loss or a breakup, your initial level of distress would likely decrease as you adapt to the new circumstances.

"People who win the coveted lottery prize experience high levels of happiness at the time. However, according to psychologists, the winners tend to return to their previous levels of happiness once the novelty of the winning experience wears off." (Corporate Finance Institute)

Interestingly, a specific study of the happiness of millionaires by Grant Donnelly and his team at Harvard Business School discovered firstly that it matters how you gained that status; if you earnt it yourself or if you inherited it. The study suggested that if you earnt the money, you would be happier. Secondly, if you have a net worth income of circa $8 million (about £6 million) you are at your happiest, in comparison to other levels of millionaires. I discuss levels of income and happiness in more detail at a later stage.

"The evolutionary task of our 'happiness module' is to improve our chances of survival and reproduction by helping us distinguish between useful and harmful, good and bad. This concept does not allow for everlasting happiness. Would the state of happiness last, we could no longer distinguish this state from others, thus losing its quality." (The Happiness Project)

Factors influencing hedonic adaptation

While hedonic adaptation occurs in most individuals, the speed and extent of adaptation can vary depending on several factors:

Duration and intensity of the event: Short-term and intense positive or negative experiences tend to result in more significant fluctuations in happiness levels initially. However, in the long run, individuals tend to adapt back to their baseline level.

Personality traits: Some individuals are naturally more resilient and predisposed to adapt more quickly to changes, both positive and negative. Traits such as optimism, emotional stability, and gratitude can influence the speed of adaptation.

Comparison and social factors: People's happiness can be influenced by their social comparisons, as they often compare their circumstances to others. This proves Aristotle's Level 2 Behaviour which is ego happiness, from comparison and doing better or being more admired by others. If individuals constantly compare themselves to others who seem to have more, they might struggle to maintain a sense of contentment, despite positive experiences.

Implications of hedonic adaptation

Understanding hedonic adaptation has several important implications for our pursuit of happiness:

Pursuit of material possessions: Hedonic adaptation challenges the notion that acquiring more material possessions or achieving certain life goals will lead to lasting happiness. It suggests that focusing on external factors alone may not bring sustained happiness. I explore this in further detail later.

Gratitude and mindfulness: Practicing gratitude and mindfulness can be effective ways to counter hedonistic adaptation. By consciously focusing on and appreciating the positive aspects of our lives, we can enhance our overall well-being. I delve into more detail on this later on.

Variety and novelty: Introducing variety and novelty into our lives can help counter the effects of adaptation. Engaging in new experiences or regularly changing our routines can provide a boost in happiness by preventing complete habituation. This is part of the reason why a holiday break is so important. Further explanation is discussed later on in the book.

Building strong relationships: Relationships and social connections play a crucial role in our overall happiness. Instead of pursuing material possessions, investing in meaningful relationships can provide a more sustained sense of satisfaction. This is covered in more detail later.

The role of genetics

It is also worth noting that while many aspects of happiness are determined by our environment and circumstances, studies have also shown that genetics play a role in our overall happiness levels. In fact, it is about 30% – 40% genetic and the rest is up to us! (Marianna Pogosyan, 2019)

However, the Body Worlds Museum in Amsterdam (The Happiness Project) suggests that it's more like 50% genetics:

"Happiness is a combination of how satisfied we are with our life and how good we feel on a day-to-day basis. It varies from person to person, but approximately 50% of our happiness is determined by genetics, 40% by our thoughts, actions and behaviours, and only 10% by circumstances (e.g. rich or poor, healthy or unhealthy, married or single)... So our actions really can make a difference."

It does seem that some people are naturally more 'happy-go-lucky' than others. I explore this in further detail later on.

Summary

The science of happiness has given us a better understanding of what makes us happy, and it can help us make conscious decisions to increase our happiness levels in the long term. While some factors such as genetics and our personal circumstances are outside our control, we can focus on practising gratitude and fostering strong social connections to boost our overall well-being. These topics are discussed in more detail later in the book.

Action time

This is a written action.

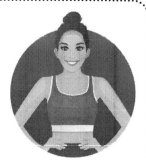

1. Using the space below, write down 5 things you are grateful for in your life at the moment. They don't all have to be huge things – it can be as simple as having a cup of your favourite tea!

2. Come back to this list when you are having a bad day to remind yourself of these 5 things.

My examples:

- I am grateful I have my health and very rarely have anything wrong with me.

- I am grateful I have a loving and understanding family support network around me.

- I am grateful I have amazing clients who appreciate what I do.

- I am grateful I have a short commute to work.

- I am grateful we have managed to book a holiday for next year.

FEEL

Balancing the triangle of life

Maintaining a balance between work, health, and family can be difficult, but it is essential for leading a fulfilling and happy life. I don't pretend to get this right all the time and I still strive for this balance. It does seem to be that when one part of this triangle is going well, another part seems to fall down spectacularly! Recently for me: boys and husband all good, work going well, but woke up with a horrible back ache for seemingly no reason. Very large sigh!

In this chapter, I explore why finding balance in these aspects of life is so crucial. Before diving in though, it's worth noting that achieving balance will differ for everyone based on individual circumstances and priorities. This chapter introduces a lot of the concepts discussed in the rest of this section of the book.

Why is finding balance with the triangle important?

Decreased stress: When we focus too much on one area of our lives, we can quickly become stressed. For example, if we put in long hours at work consistently without taking breaks, this can lead to burnout, impacting our physical and mental health. Consequently, finding a balance between work and personal life can significantly reduce stress levels.

Improved relationships: Neglecting our family and social relationships can create tension and may impact our emotional well-being. While putting in long hours at work, we may become isolated from our loved ones and/or have no time for them. It is, therefore, beneficial to make time for family and friends regularly. I absolutely love the idea below from Harvard University about needing to exercise relationships in the same way we keep our bodies fit and working properly:

"To make sure your relationships are healthy and balanced, it's important to practice 'social fitness.' We tend to think that once we

establish friendships and intimate relationships, they will take care of themselves. But our social life is a living system, and it needs exercise." (CNBC.com discussing Harvard University Happiness study)

Better health: When we neglect our health, our overall well-being is affected, potentially leading to anxiety, stress, and illness. Physical exercise, a balanced diet, and sufficient sleep are essential components to maintain good health, ensuring higher productivity levels. These topics are covered in much more detail in later sections of this book.

To achieve a proper balance between work, family, and health, the following strategies may help. Each of these are also covered in more detail in further sections of this book.

Prioritise and schedule: It's crucial to clarify what matters most and prioritise accordingly. Then, schedule and allocate time to these areas of life. Be specific with scheduling what time and how much you'll dedicate to work, family, and health per day, week, or month.

Learn to break away from work: When working remotely and with technology advancements, it is easy to check work emails and notifications 24/7. Building habits to disconnect from work can promote mental relaxation, and improve overall happiness. Put your laptop and phone down, and have a chat with the family!

Learn to say no: It can be challenging to say no on occasion, but it is essential. For instance, taking on too much work can lead to a skewed balance between health, work, and family. So, understand your workload capacities and say no to tasks that exceed your workload. I am absolutely terrible at this and need to learn the benefits of using this tool more often – so if you are my client or colleague reading this book, sorry in advance!!

Make time for yourself: Carve out a little bit of time each day to do something that makes you feel good, whether it's reading a book, taking a walk, meditating, or watching your favourite programme with a cup of tea. Keep in mind that this time is solely for you – not easy to do with a busy schedule, but super important.

"Unless you have the most varied and interesting job in the world, then you're only going to be a one-dimensional human being if you never come outside of it. Please don't be boring! Fresh perspectives gained from interests, hobbies, and outside reading are going to make you better at your work-life and relationship-balanced life. You will have more creative and diverse ways to think about what you do, which makes for better output." (Paul Richlovsky)

Prioritise sleep: The amount and quality of your sleep can greatly affect your mood, productivity, and ability to handle stress. You must be able to remember the negative feelings and lack of productivity you experienced the last time you didn't get enough sleep. Create a regular sleep schedule and try to go to bed and wake up at the same time every day if you can.

Practice mindfulness: Mindfulness is the practice of being present and aware of your thoughts, feelings, and surroundings. You can incorporate mindfulness in your daily routine by taking deep breaths, focusing on your senses, or journaling your thoughts.

Exercise regularly: As a PT, I may be a little biased, but not only is it good for your physical health to exercise, it can also help relieve stress and improve your mood. Aim for at least 30 minutes minimum of physical activity every day, even if this is simply a walk around the block.

Seek social support: Having a supportive network of friends or family members can help alleviate stress, give you encouragement, and make you feel loved. If you have had a rubbish day, it will always help to ring your bestie and have a good natter!

Summary

Work, health, and family are essential areas of life, and achieving balance can be difficult. However, the benefits that come with finding balance despite challenges are numerous. In essence, health should be the most prioritised, followed by family, then work. Take steps to schedule, prioritise, say no, and break away when applicable to ensure that these areas of life are kept in proper balance.

Action Time

This is a practical action.

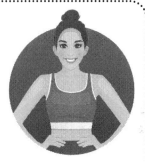

1. Try stopping work and putting your computer/tools down every Friday at 5 pm on the dot, each week for a whole month.

2. At 5:01 pm, grab the dog and go for a 30-minute walk before starting your weekend. Or if you don't own a dog – simply go for a walk!

3. Do you feel better? I bet you do!

My example: I don't finish work in the gym until around 9 pm most weekday evenings due to PT sessions, but I do usually get an hour or so break in the middle of the day. I will get home, eat something, then take Teddy (our little Cavapoo) out for a walk, usually with my husband (he works from home a lot so needs the break as well). It's a fabulous way to break up the day, get some fresh air, and provide the dog with some well-needed exercise. I may not have a nine-to-five job, but trying to find balance is still vital.

Cultivating gratitude

"Research shows gratitude isn't just a pleasant feeling – being grateful can also support greater health, happiness, and wisdom in ourselves and our communities." (mindful.org)

In a world overwhelmed by negativity and challenges, it becomes essential to cultivate gratitude and appreciate the good in life. Gratitude is a powerful practice that has the ability to shift our perspective, enhance our overall well-being, and bring us closer to a state of happiness. This isn't easy though, especially if it seems as if multiple things are going wrong at the same time! In this chapter, we explore the importance of gratitude, practical ways to introduce it into our daily lives, and how appreciating the positive aspects of life can lead us to a happier and more fulfilling existence.

The power of gratitude

Gratitude is the act of acknowledging and appreciating the good things we have in our lives, big or small. It provides a shift in mindset that allows us to focus on what we do have rather than what we lack. Research suggests that cultivating gratitude has numerous benefits, including increased happiness, improved mental health, strengthened relationships, and enhanced resilience.

"Gratitude is strongly and consistently associated with greater happiness. Gratitude helps people feel more positive emotions, relish good experiences, improve their health, deal with adversity, and build strong relationships." (Harvard Health Publishing, 2021)

Practising gratitude daily

Developing a habit of practising gratitude is crucial to reap its benefits fully. This takes some practice if you are not used to it. Here are a few practical ways to incorporate gratitude into your daily routine:

Gratitude journal: Set aside a few minutes each day to write down three things you are grateful for. Be specific and reflect on the reasons that brought you joy or appreciation in those moments. This habit helps train your brain to focus on the positives. To give you an example; today I am grateful that my back ache feels much better, that I had a productive week at work, and that my son had a great weekend karting.

Gratitude walks: When you get a chance, take a leisurely stroll outdoors and pay attention to the beauty around you. Notice the colours of flowers, the chirping of birds, or the warmth of sunlight. Engaging your senses and expressing gratitude for these simple pleasures can bring immense joy. This is covered later on in more detail.

Gratitude letters: Write a heartfelt letter to someone you are grateful for in your life. Express your appreciation clearly for their presence, support, or their positive impact on you. The art of writing or receiving a letter is lost in today's modern life – this makes it even more special. The other day, I wrote a gratitude letter for a friend who was moving countries – let's just say we both cried (with joy); it was very sweet!

"In one study involving nearly 300 adults seeking counselling services at a university, one randomized group wrote a gratitude letter each week for three weeks. The gratitude group reported significantly better mental health (compared to the control group) at follow-up, 12 weeks after the last writing exercise. Another type of written gratitude practice is counting blessings, or 'Three Good Things.' A study of this practice found that people who wrote down three things that had gone well in their day and identified the causes of those good things were

significantly happier and less depressed, even six months after the study ended. " (mindful.org)

Shifting perspective

Appreciating the good in life often requires a shift in perspective. It involves focusing on the positive aspects, even amidst challenges. Here are some strategies to help you change your perspective:

Gratitude in adversity: During difficult times, make an effort to find something positive or a lesson you have learned. This might be an opportunity for personal growth or a chance to appreciate the strength and resilience you possess. I appreciate this is not an easy task, especially depending on the circumstances you are in. Being potentially controversial, I often find a loved one's funeral an opportunity to reflect and practice gratitude. It helps to think further about how the deceased enriched your life and what you would like to add or change in your future. This point is discussed in more detail later in the book.

Mindful moments: Engage in mindfulness practices to bring your attention to the present moment. Notice the sensations, thoughts, and emotions that arise. In these moments, reflect on the abundance of good things that surround you, no matter how small. Only today I found myself engaging in mindfulness; it was a particularly sunny, warm day today (rare, I know!!) and I was working indoors, but when I went outside, I stood still for a few moments, listened to the world, soaked up the sun, and breathed in and out slowly and peacefully. It was only a few moments before I had to get back to work, but it was beautiful.

Avoid comparison: Comparing yourself to others can reduce the ability to appreciate the good in our lives. Remember that everyone's journey is unique and focusing on your own blessings can prevent feelings of envy or inadequacy. In the fitness industry, in particular, this is rife! It is very easy to look at others on social media, for example, and want to be like them or look like them. It is important to understand that everything is not always as it seems, and remember that you are on your **own** journey, not theirs.

Building gratitude in relationships

Gratitude can strengthen our connections with others and foster a positive environment. Here's how you can utilise gratitude to deepen your relationships:

Expressing appreciation: Regularly express your gratitude to loved ones, friends, and co-workers. A simple thank you or acknowledging someone's efforts can create a ripple effect of positivity. If you hold a managerial position at work, please remember this will make a world of difference to the positivity and productivity of your team.

Gratitude rituals: Create rituals within your relationships to highlight gratitude. For example, during family meals, take turns sharing something each person is grateful for that day. This practice can instil a sense of unity and appreciation among everyone involved.

Random acts of kindness: This is a popular topic on social media at the moment. Perform small acts of kindness for others without expecting anything in return. This could be as simple as holding the door for someone, leaving a thoughtful note, or offering help when needed. These acts not only benefit others but also foster a sense of gratitude within ourselves. The Random Acts of Kindness Foundation (how brilliant!!) wrote a great article on the Science of Kindness stating that it reduces your stress levels, referencing the study below:

"Perpetually kind people have 23% less cortisol (the stress hormone) and age slower than the average population!" (McCraty et al, 1998)

Summary

Cultivating gratitude and appreciating the good in life is a transformative practice that can lead to a more fulfilled and happy existence. By incorporating gratitude into our daily routines, shifting our perspectives, and nurturing relationships, we can unlock the power of gratitude and embrace the abundance that surrounds us. Start today and watch as this practice brings positive changes to every aspect of your life.

Action Time

This is a written action.

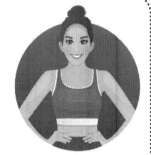

1. Using the space on the next page, write down as many ideas as you can, to be kind to someone else. This could be a family member, someone at work, a neighbour, or a friend.

2. Next, narrow this down to your two best acts of kindness. What exactly would you do and why would you do it? Be specific.

3. Make a pact with yourself that you are going to do these two acts.

4. Plan when you are going to do them, then go for it.

5. Note down how you felt afterwards. Feeling great?! I thought so ☺

My example: My sister has been feeling mentally exhausted recently and could do with a fun day out where she is not focused on the daily grind. My act of kindness is to take her out for a fun and relaxing afternoon tea (something she loves doing!) in a new location she hasn't been to before as a lovely treat and surprise. It is only a small gesture, but she will really appreciate it and this in turn will make me feel very happy to do this for her.

Watch out: happiness is catching!

"Research shows that close contact with a happy person increases our chance of being happy by 15%." (The Happiness Project)

We have all met both these sets of people in life: the 'glass half full' and the 'glass half empty' people! Who would you rather be in a meeting with, have lunch with, or get stuck in the lift with? Outwardly showing and sharing your happiness is infectious! But why is this the case?

As a rule, human beings are social creatures, born with an innate tendency to seek connections and interact with others. Our interactions with different individuals throughout our lives significantly impact our emotions, thoughts, and overall well-being. In this chapter, we will explore the science behind why being a happy person positively affects others around you.

The brain's mirror neurons

One crucial aspect of understanding our preference for positive individuals lies in the existence of mirror neurons within our brain. Mirror neurons are specialised cells that become active not only when we perform a particular action, but also when we observe someone else performing it. These neurons play a significant role in the human ability to empathise and connect with others on an emotional level. Mirror neurons are at play, for instance, when you are in a meeting and you find yourself copying another person's actions – leaning forward, leaning on hands, cupping your face, pushing your hair back, and so on. Not that you know it at the time, but you are trying to connect with each other by copying each other's actions.

When we encounter positive, happy individuals, our mirror neurons become activated, mirroring their emotions within our own brain. This mirroring subsequently elicits positive emotions within ourselves, resulting in an uplifting effect on our mood. This is why we are naturally drawn to positive people – they have the ability to inspire and boost our own well-being through the simple act of being happy.

Let me give you an example. Has someone, who is perhaps a naturally negative person, said to you, "Are you OK today? You look tired and not too well. I'm not feeling great today either..."? Immediately, you feel tired and not too well, even if you were feeling fine! And the opposite is also true. Passing conversation from a positive, upbeat person such as, "Ooooh, you are looking fabulous today! Loving the dress!", you immediately feel good about yourself and ready to tackle the day!

I read a fascinating article in Forbes when researching this part of the book referencing the Framingham Heart Study by N.A. Christakis at Harvard in 2008. I loved this idea of happiness being something infectious that spreads:

"You've heard of six degrees of separation: the idea that all people are connected to each other within six or less social connections. Happiness is similarly connected. Based on the study of 5,000 people over 20 years, when an individual is happy, the feeling tends to spread through three degrees of separation. So, if your colleague is happy, the positivity will spill over to three others. In contrast, sadness did not seem to have this spreading effect." (forbes.com)

The impact on our physiology

As previously discussed, research has shown that positive emotions, such as happiness, can lead to the release of various neurotransmitters and hormones that contribute to our overall well-being.

Endorphins: Positive interactions with happy people can trigger the release of endorphins in our brain. Endorphins – often referred to as 'feel-good' chemicals – act as natural painkillers and play a vital role in reducing stress, promoting relaxation, and fostering a sense of positivity.

Serotonin: Another crucial neurotransmitter influenced by positive social interactions is serotonin. Increased serotonin levels are associated with improved mood, emotional stability, and a decreased risk of developing mental health issues such as depression and anxiety.

Immune System Boost: Studies have shown that positive emotions can boost your immune system. During happy and positive encounters, the body's production of antibodies and other immune cells increases, enhancing our ability to ward off infections and providing better overall protection against diseases.

"The specific physiological responses induced by pleasant stimuli were recently investigated with the immune and endocrine systems being monitored when pleasant stimuli such as odours and emotional pictures were presented to subjects. The results revealed that an increase in secretory immunoglobulin A and a decrease in salivary cortisol were induced by pleasant emotions." (sciencedirect.com)

Mental and emotional well-being

The effects of surrounding ourselves with positive, happy individuals extend beyond the physical state of our bodies. Our mental and emotional well-being also benefit greatly.

Stress reduction: Positive social connections can act as a significant buffer against stress. Interacting with positive people promotes feelings of optimism, reducing stress levels and improving the overall quality of our lives.

Emotional resilience: Being around positive people can improve our emotional resilience, allowing us to cope better with challenging situations. Observing their positive outlook, we learn to develop more optimistic perspectives, which in turn helps us navigate difficulties with increased courage and resilience.

Expanded social support: Surrounding ourselves with positive individuals tends to create an environment that fosters a strong social support system. This mutual support network bolsters our sense of belonging, enhances our self-esteem, and reduces feelings of isolation or loneliness.

Positive mindset forming

So if it is best for us to seek out positivity, how can we do this and how can we be there for others around us? It's all about positive mindset forming. One of the most well-known theories regarding a positive mindset is the 'cup half full vs. cup half empty' mindset.

The 'cup half full' mentality is based on the idea that, in any situation, there is always a silver lining. This mindset focuses on the positive aspects of any given situation, rather than dwelling on the negative. It's about seeing the positive in things and striving to find solutions rather than feeling stuck in a problem.

On the other hand, the 'cup half empty' mentality is based on a negative outlook. This mindset focuses on the negative aspects of any situation and tends to highlight the problems rather than the solutions. It's about being pessimistic and feeling stuck rather than working towards a resolution.

When it comes to developing a positive mindset, it is important to recognise that the way we perceive things is entirely up to us, and we can choose to see things in a positive light, even during challenging times. We can reframe our thoughts from negative to positive, and this will have a significant impact on our mental state.

I'm not saying this is easy, however, so here are some tips to help cultivate a 'cup half full' mindset:

Focus on gratitude: Instead of focusing on what you lack, try to appreciate the things you have and the people in your life who support you. For example, I'm glad the sun is shining today and my kids have gone back to school!

Practice positive self-talk: Be kind to yourself and embrace positive affirmations. Remind yourself daily of your strengths and accomplishments. For example, I have just completed a workout at the gym and I am so pleased that I managed to get myself there. Good for me!

Surround yourself with positivity: Surrounding yourself with positive people and uplifting messages can help keep you in a positive frame of mind. For example, I have this minute sent one of my best friends a message wishing him a productive and positive day as he has meetings in London all day. He will receive this message, smile, and it will put him in a more positive frame of mind.

Look for the good in every situation: Even in challenging situations, look for the silver lining and try to reframe your thoughts into something positive. For example, my child is being very annoying right now as he is getting frustrated, waiting for us to finish work before we go and do a task together. The positive side of this is at least he wants to do something with us and is willing to help us with the task.

Let go of negative self-talk: Negative self-talk can hold us back from achieving our goals. Instead, focus on the positive and replace negative self-talk with positive affirmations. For example, I try not to say "I can't." Instead, I try to say "I can't … yet."

Summary

The science is clear: our preference for positive, happy people is grounded in the physiology of our brains and the impact they have on our bodies and minds, and having a positive mindset can help lead to a more fulfilling and happy life. Surrounding ourselves with 'cup half full' people not only lifts our spirits but also improves our overall well-being. By understanding the underlying mechanisms, we can actively cultivate and seek out positive, happy individuals to nourish our own happiness and that of others.

Action Time

This is a practical action.

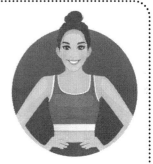

1. Next time you are sitting with colleagues, having a break or waiting for a meeting to start, mention something positive that has happened to you recently.

2. Notice the response. It's very likely to be positive and they may well start talking about something positive too!

3. If you are not in meetings often, try it at home with your immediate family.

My example: I was waiting for everyone to arrive to a meeting so we could commence. Simply asking what people got up to at the weekend and saying that I was pleased with how well I had tackled some DIY, started a whole positive chat on painting, decorating and home improvements around the meeting table. The positive atmosphere had a big impact on the meeting itself, which was productive and fun.

The power of laughter

"Everybody loves to laugh! In fact, adults laugh on average 17 times per day, and children up to 400 times!" (The Happiness Project)

"Laughter is the best medicine. It not only heals others, but also helps lighten our daily loads, and brings a smile to our face and everyone we meet." (Heggie, 2019)

Laughter is an extraordinary human ability that has the power to transform lives. We all know the saying 'laughter is the best medicine', and its benefits extend far beyond a simple moment of amusement. Think of your favourite comedian or comedy shows and how you feel after watching a few of their sketches – they have a very important job to do.

One of my favourite comedies has to be the BBC *Blackadder* series (yes, I am showing my age now!) – so quotable and still very funny even over 30 years later!

Dr Johnson: *Here it is, sire. A very cornerstone of English scholarship. This book contains every word in our beloved language.*

Blackadder: *Every single one, sir?*

Dr Johnson: *Every single one, sir.*

Blackadder: *In that case, sir, I hope you will not object if I also offer the Doctor my most enthusiastic contrafibularities.*

Dr Johnson: *What, sir?*

Blackadder: *Contrafibularities, sir. It is a common word down our way.*

Dr Johnson: *Damn!*

Blackadder: *Oh, I'm sorry, sir. I am anaspeptic, phrasmodic, even compunctuous to have caused you such periconbobulations.*

(Blackadder the Third, episode 2)

In this chapter, we will explore the profound impact that laughter can have on our physical, mental, and emotional well-being, as well as its ability to build connections and bring joy to our lives.

The physical benefits of laughter

Laughter not only feels good, but also produces positive physiological changes in our bodies. When we laugh, our brain releases endorphins, which are natural feel-good chemicals that can help reduce stress and pain. Additionally, laughter stimulates our heart and respiratory systems, resulting in increased oxygen flow and improved cardiovascular health. Studies have shown that regular laughter can even strengthen our immune system, making us more resilient to illnesses.

"Short term benefits include stimulating your heart, lungs and muscles, activates and relieves your stress response, and soothes tension. Long term benefits include improving your immune system, pain relief, increase personal satisfaction, and improved mood." (Mayo Clinic, 2023)

"Laughter triggers healthy physical changes in our body. Humour and laughter strengthen our immune system, boost our energy, diminish pain, and protect us from the damaging effects of stress. Best of all, this priceless medicine is fun, free and easy to use." (The Happiness Project)

The mental and emotional impact

Laughter has tremendous mental and emotional benefits. It reduces feelings of anxiety and depression by promoting the release of neurotransmitters like dopamine and serotonin, which are known to boost mood and enhance overall mental well-being. By reducing stress levels, laughter can improve cognitive function, memory, and creativity. Moreover, it helps us gain perspective, shift our mindset, and approach challenges with a lighter attitude.

Social bonding through laughter

"Share a laugh! Spreading laughter is the next best thing to laughing yourself. When laughter is shared, it binds people together and increases happiness and intimacy." (The Happiness Project)

Laughter is a powerful tool for building connections and strengthening relationships. When we share a hearty laugh with others, it creates a sense of belonging and fosters camaraderie. Laughter can break down barriers, diffuse tension and conflicts, and provide a shared positive experience. It also helps build trust, as it signals to others that we are approachable, friendly, and capable of seeing the lighter side of life. Of course, certain situations do call for more reflective contemplation, concentration, and a more serious tone, but next time you find yourself in a meeting that could potentially be very dull, if appropriate, try adding in a bit of humour. I have done this many times in meetings and it's a great ice-breaker and relaxes the attendees.

The healing power of laughter

Laughter can be a transformative force in difficult situations, providing comfort and healing even in the face of adversity. It acts as a coping mechanism, helping individuals to find solace amidst pain or grief. Laughter promotes resilience and enables us to bounce back from life's hardships by offering moments of respite and a fresh perspective. It allows us to maintain hope, find joy, and move forward with renewed strength. The analogy below made me smile for sure:

"Laughter brings physiological benefits to the body. It lessens people's pain, so if anything, we need to be spreading more healing laughter in all of our interactions. It is like a bee pollinating flowers and bringing them to life." (Heggie, 2019)

It is all relative, but if I find myself having a bad day where it seems that nothing has gone to plan, I can either cry about it, or laugh. Laughing is definitely the best medicine! I have a number of clients that make me laugh all the time and we often share a few silly moments together whilst training.

Summary

Laughter is not simply a fleeting moment of amusement; it has a profound impact on our physical, mental, and emotional well-being. Its ability to strengthen the immune system, reduce stress, enhance mood, and foster social connections is simply remarkable. By embracing laughter, we can reap its numerous benefits and improve our overall quality of life. So, let us not underestimate the power of laughter – let us laugh wholeheartedly, share in its joy, and spread its healing effects to make the world a brighter place.

Action Time

This is a practical action.

Dad jokes! Still funny and quite innocent most of the time.

1. Look up a selection of jokes on the internet.

2. Pick your favourites and have a good old laugh!

My examples:

"My boss told me to have a good day. So, I went home."

"What's the friendliest cheese? Halloumi."

My 11-year-old son and I do this on occasion – and it's even more funny when you have to explain the joke when he doesn't 'get it'!!

Anti-happiness

They say 'every cloud has a silver lining' – this chapter looks at the 'cloud' a bit more.

Unfortunately, you can't be happy all the time, so what is your body doing when you are feeling 'blue'? When humans experience negative emotions such as sadness, there are a number of different chemical reactions that occur in the brain. While these chemical reactions are complex and varied, here are a few key ones that help explain why we feel sad:

Decreased serotonin levels: Serotonin is a neurotransmitter that helps regulate mood, appetite, and sleep. When serotonin levels drop, we may experience feelings of sadness or anxiety. This is why some medications that boost serotonin levels, such as selective serotonin reuptake inhibitors (SSRIs), are used to treat depression.

Increased cortisol levels: Cortisol is a hormone that is released in response to stress. Elevated cortisol levels can contribute to feelings of tension, anxiety, and sadness over time. Chronic stress can also lead to changes in brain structure and function that can further worsen mood.

Changes in dopamine signalling: Dopamine is a neurotransmitter that is involved in reward and pleasure processing. When we experience something pleasurable, our brains release dopamine, which helps us feel good. However, when we're feeling sad, dopamine signalling can be disrupted. This can contribute to a sense of apathy or lack of motivation.

Disrupted neural pathways: Negative emotions, such as sadness, can cause changes in brain circuitry over time. For example, chronic stress can damage and shrink the hippocampus part of the brain, which is involved in memory and emotion regulation.

So what makes us feel sad? There are a number of reasons why we might feel down, including:

- Life events: Sadness can be a natural response to a major life event, such as the loss of a loved one or the end of a relationship.

- Biological factors: Some people may be more predisposed to depression or other mood disorders due to genetic or environmental factors.

- Chronic stress: Stress can take a toll on our bodies and minds, leading to feelings of sadness or anxiety.

- Lack of social support: Humans are social animals. When we lack social support, we may be more prone to negative emotions.

The Happiness Project in the Body Worlds Museum in Amsterdam explains very clearly what happens to us when we try to deal with the strains of modern life. Below is an extract from the exhibition. It explains that we need the stress hormones in our body but if they are constantly being overused, then it can cause us harm:

"Stress impacts our mental and physical well-being in either positive or negative ways.

When experiencing stress or danger, the entire body is in a heightened state of alertness due to increased levels of cortisol and adrenaline. The hormones trigger a chain of symptoms: elevated heart rate and blood pressure, heavier breathing and sweating. At the same time, glucose reserves are tapped to provide the body with more energy.

Moderate stress, small bursts of energy from an adrenaline rush, give us a sense of well-being. It can improve memory, strengthen our immune system, prepare us for difficult tasks, and boost productivity.

However, the demands of modern life are leaving one in four of us permanently stressed. Over time, the powerful stress hormones coursing through our bodies cripple our immune system and compromise our health. Continued (chronic) stress can raise blood pressure, increase the risk of heart attack and stroke, increase vulnerability to anxiety and depression, contribute to infertility, and hasten the ageing process.

An absence of stress, on the other hand, can result in a lack of motivation, and feelings of boredom, lethargy, or depression."

Overcoming obstacles and dealing with setbacks

Life is filled with obstacles, setbacks, and challenges that can often lead us to feel discouraged, overwhelmed and certainly not happy. However, it is essential to remember that these obstacles are not roadblocks, but opportunities for growth and resilience.

I would like to share a very personal story with you about a three-day period that happened very recently, just before this book got published. For the first time in my life, I felt completely overwhelmed and experienced physical symptoms because of it. I am usually someone who can tolerate high levels of stress and am a multi-tasker who thrives on having lots of activities going on at the same time. But sometimes the stress-funnel of life gets filled up too much and even the strongest of people can get completely overwhelmed and are not able to cope.

Here is the what happened in three days, in no particular order, and this is on top of usual workload. I am, unfortunately, not exaggerating for the purposes of effect – this all really happened:

- My eldest son had a bad karting accident, broke his arm and had to have emergency surgery

- My youngest son hurt his foot at football and he couldn't walk properly for two days. It wasn't broken but was badly bruised

- I completed a six-hour walking competition and in the process pulled my right glute muscle, so was struggling with the pain

- My husband was away with work in a different country so couldn't really help

- My parents were away on holiday in a different country and they don't tend to look at their phones

- My sister was at a client work site hours away and couldn't really communicate

- My kids had an inset day from school so I had to juggle work and looking after them – they don't get on at all and it is quite stressful leaving them at home together

- One of my dearest friends, whom I love very much, is experiencing huge problems at work and home. They decided to take it out on me and were extremely hurtful and cold towards me, and certainly didn't have the capacity to help me at all

- A PT client had to quit on me because they were made redundant

- Two PT clients said they are going to struggle to commit to sessions with me for much longer due to financial constraints

- One PT client who was due to be coming back after maternity leave decided against it

- After consultations with three potential PT clients, they all decided to leave it for now, due to financial constraints

- Our house went 'under offer' and we don't have anywhere to move to yet

- I organise a team for an annual sporting event and it's great fun, but very time-consuming. One by one they all had to quit, only a few days before the event. One was my transport to the event, so I couldn't do it either

- I missed a magazine print deadline because my designer didn't get back to me in time with the final artwork

- We were supposed to hear about a pitch for a new gym but the client missed the deadline to let us know, so we are still none the wiser

- Due to being in hospital with one child overnight, and my stress levels on the other two nights, I had a total sum of 10 hours' sleep in three days.

The effect of these three days meant that for the first time I got upset at work, something I never do. I tried very hard not to show it in front of clients, but I certainly had to showcase my best acting skills. When I got home, I completely shut down; I felt very cold, could hardly walk and nearly fainted, felt sick, couldn't eat anything, couldn't talk, couldn't stop staring into space, and couldn't comprehend what anyone was saying to me. This lasted all day. My stress funnel was overflowing and there was nothing I could see to do about it at the time. Even with all the coping mechanisms that I have been taught and practice, I still couldn't stop this from happening.

Conclusion: There is only a certain amount that I can cope with; I am not Superwoman.

What were my learnings from these three days? Firstly, I needed to remember that this amount of chaos and negativity very rarely happens to me so I am unlikely to have this again for a while. Secondly, my support group did come back from being away and were there to help straight after this happened – in addition, they are usually there for me. Thirdly, it reinforced how you can't be in control of every aspect of your life, so you need to try very hard to let the small things go and prioritise. It also really helped me to build resilience for potential future obstacles.

Developing a resilient mindset

Building resilience is crucial for overcoming obstacles. Although not easy at all, here are some key principles to adopt:

Embracing failure as a learning opportunity: Reframe failure as a stepping-stone towards success rather than a limitation. Learn from mistakes, analyse what went wrong, and use this knowledge to improve your approach.

Cultivating a growth mindset: Adopt a belief that your abilities and intelligence can be developed through dedication and hard work. Embrace challenges as opportunities to grow and enhance your skills, knowing that effort and perseverance can lead to improvement.

Maintaining a positive attitude: Approach setbacks with optimism and a belief that there is a solution or lesson hidden within them. Reframe difficulties as temporary hurdles that can be overcome through determination and resilience.

Is it resilience rather than happiness?

When researching the resilient mind for this book, I started to wonder whether when we view something as happiness, could it be resilience instead? Resilience is the capacity to bounce back, to regain strength, and to develop adaptable coping mechanisms in the face of adversity. It is not about being immune to pain or avoiding difficulties, but rather about embracing a mindset that allows us to view challenges as opportunities for growth.

Resilience encourages us to shift our focus from constantly seeking happiness to learning how to cope effectively with the wide range of experiences life throws our way. It teaches us that happiness can be found not only in joyous occasions, but also in moments of struggle, learning, and self-discovery.

The Tao of coping

The ancient Chinese philosophy of Taoism emphasises the importance of embracing the natural flow of life's events, both positive and negative. Taoism teaches us to relinquish control and accept the reality of impermanence. By developing resilience, we adopt the Taoist perspective and learn to 'roll with the punches', finding strength in flexibility and adaptability.

"By letting it go it all gets done. The world is won by those who let it go. But when you try and try. The world is beyond the winning."

Lao Tzu (6th century BC – 5th century BC)
Ancient Chinese Taoist philosopher

Psychological resilience factors

Psychologists have identified several key factors that contribute to the development of resilience. These factors include:

Positive mindset: Cultivating an optimistic outlook and reframing challenges as opportunities for growth can enhance resilience. By focusing on solutions rather than dwelling on problems, we can develop a proactive approach to life.

Social support: Building strong and meaningful connections with others provides a vital foundation for resilience. A network of supportive relationships can offer encouragement, guidance, and a sense of belonging during difficult times.

Emotional regulation: Learning to manage our emotions and exercise self-control allows us to navigate challenging situations more effectively. By developing emotional intelligence, we can regulate our responses and maintain a balanced state of mind.

Self-reflection and adaptability: Resilience requires self-awareness and the willingness to learn from our experiences. By reflecting on our actions and attitudes, we can adapt and grow, strengthening our ability to overcome adversity.

The resilient mindset

Resilience is not a one-time achievement; it is an ongoing process that requires continuous effort and self-reflection. By cultivating a resilient mindset, we can embrace life's uncertainties and learn to cope with whatever comes our way. This mindset involves:

- Embracing change: Recognising that change is inevitable allows us to let go of the need for control and adapt to life's fluctuations.

- Practising gratitude: Appreciating the present moment and acknowledging the positive aspects of our lives can help us find joy even during challenging times.

- Seeking growth: Embracing challenges as opportunities for personal growth allows us to develop the skills and wisdom needed to overcome difficulties.

- Building resilience habits: Engaging in regular self-care practices, such as exercise, mindfulness, and seeking support when needed, helps to strengthen our resilience over time.

In the very practical and useful book *Resilient* by Rick Hanson, they discuss the idea of needing a good dose of grit. *"Grit is about being tough and resourceful... it's the feeling that you can make things happen in the world, instead of helplessly going with the flow."* Another concept discussed is that we will be more resilient if we learn to stay calm about situations. *"...we have a tendency to overestimate threats, whilst also underestimating our ability to handle them. The result? A lot of anxiety that serves no useful function and drains us of the energy we need to face real problems."*

While happiness may come and go, resilience empowers us to find contentment and joy amidst life's trials and tribulations. By adopting a resilient mindset, learning to cope effectively, and viewing challenges as opportunities for growth, we can forge a path towards lasting happiness and fulfilment.

Strategies for overcoming obstacles

Another aspect of 'anti-happiness' is the constant need for us to overcome obstacles put in our path. When faced with obstacles, having effective strategies to overcome them is essential. Here are a few techniques to help you tackle challenges head-on:

Break it down: Identify the specific components of the obstacle or challenge, and break it down into manageable tasks. By taking small steps, you can work towards overcoming the obstacle one piece at a time, reducing feelings of overwhelm. We have been taught this since primary school age: in Maths, break down the problem and show your workings out to get to the final answer. When writing an English essay, start with your introduction, have a few main points you can back up with evidence, and then make sure you add a conclusion.

Seek support and guidance: Reach out to trusted friends, mentors, or professionals who can provide advice, guidance, or emotional support. They may offer fresh perspectives and new ideas, or act as a sounding board for brainstorming solutions. This is one of the reasons clients sign up to work with me! We are not meant to know everything – seek advice and answers from others more experienced and qualified than you.

Adapt and adjust: Be flexible and open to adjusting your approach or strategy when faced with obstacles. Sometimes, a change in perspective or a willingness to adapt can lead to breakthroughs.

Managing setbacks

Setbacks are inevitable along the path towards success. Here are some strategies to help you manage setbacks effectively:

Acknowledge and accept emotions: Allow yourself to feel and process the emotions associated with setbacks, such as frustration, disappointment, or sadness. Ignoring or suppressing these emotions can hinder your ability to bounce back. Give yourself time and space to reflect before moving forward.

Reframe setbacks: See setbacks as opportunities for growth, learning, and self-improvement. Look for the lessons embedded within setbacks and view them as stepping-stones towards future success.

Practice self-compassion: Treat yourself with kindness and understanding during setbacks. Avoid self-blame and negative self-talk. Remind yourself that setbacks are a natural part of life, and success often emerges from these moments of adversity.

Can you find happiness in the bleakest of situations?

It may seem challenging to find happiness in the bleakest of situations, such as war or a terminal illness. However, happiness and contentment can be found even in the midst of extreme adversity. Below I explore the idea that happiness is not solely dependent on external circumstances, but can be cultivated through inner strength, perspective, and embracing the present moment.

Cultivating inner strength

Finding happiness in bleak situations requires cultivating inner strength. It involves developing resilience, gratitude, and a sense of purpose.

Resilience in war: During war, individuals may find strength in their commitment to their beliefs and values. By focusing on noble causes, they can find a sense of purpose and a higher meaning, which can contribute to happiness even in the midst of chaos.

Resilience in terminal illness: Those facing terminal illness might find strength through acceptance, emotional support, and unconditional love from loved ones. Embracing the present moment, creating meaningful connections, and finding joy in small moments can contribute to happiness even during challenging times.

Shifting perspective

Perspective plays a vital role in finding happiness even in bleak situations. By intentionally shifting our perspective, we can find light in the darkness. Here are a few strategies:

Finding beauty in small pleasures: In turbulent times or illness, finding joy in simple pleasures can bring happiness. Appreciating a beautiful sunset, a meaningful conversation, or acts of kindness can shift the focus from despair to gratitude.

Redefining success and happiness: Rethinking the traditional definition of success and happiness is crucial in challenging situations. By focusing on inner growth, personal connections, and acts of kindness, individuals can find fulfilment regardless of external circumstances.

Despite the unimaginable circumstances of war and terminal illness, stories of happiness can be found:

In the midst of conflict, individuals often find happiness in camaraderie with fellow soldiers, fighting for a cause they believe in, or experiencing moments of peace amidst chaos. Acts of bravery, resilience, and the pursuit of justice can bring a sense of purpose and fulfilment.

Spike Milligan's *Adolf Hitler: My Part in His Downfall* was written in the middle of a war zone. Although the topic is sombre and tragic, Spike still managed to find moments of joy, laughter, and pleasure. A good example of how durable and persistent happiness can be.

Facing a terminal illness can lead individuals to discover a new-found appreciation for life. By cherishing and deeply experiencing moments with loved ones, finding peace in spiritual beliefs, and focusing on personal growth, individuals can find happiness even in the face of mortality.

I spoke to a couple of my clients who happen to be hospital doctors (frequently in A&E and ICU units) and I was curious to understand if they have experienced joy and happiness from patients in a critical situation. I was very surprised to hear that it happens all the time! Even when in hospital with one of my children recently, there were some extremely unwell children in the ward, but there was plenty of laughter, energy, and positivity from staff and the children themselves. I was genuinely very surprised to experience first-hand the level of happiness that can come from such trauma.

One of my friends recently described a story that exemplifies this further. His best friend recently passed away from breast cancer, but when she first was told of her diagnosis and prognosis (which wasn't positive at all), instead of falling into despair, she felt a sense of relief and inner peace that she knew what was going to happen. She had time to plan, sort her affairs, and say goodbye to people properly. The little things that would worry others were no stress or consequence anymore, and she kept her sense of humour right until the end, including her funeral, in which she had a full say. None of us will ever know what we would do or feel like if faced with this situation ourselves, and although I didn't know this lady personally, I think she was a complete inspiration to everyone around her and hopefully to you as well, dear reader.

There are several writers, including Viktor E. Frankl, the noted Austrian neurologist, psychiatrist and Holocaust survivor, who state that happiness cannot be truly understood and appreciated, or indeed even felt, if suffering has never been felt before, as there is no comparison. I think that's a difficult concept to fully comprehend because I would argue it is all relative. If I haven't been through a horrific situation, does that mean that I cannot truly comprehend or experience true happiness?

"There is often a complex and dynamic relationship between happiness and suffering. There is a Chinese saying: 'The extreme form of happiness produces sorrow'. Just as happiness may lead to suffering, so does suffering lead to happiness."

Dr Paul Wong
Canadian psychologist

Summary

Overcoming obstacles and dealing with setbacks is an integral part of any meaningful journey. By developing a resilient mindset, adopting effective strategies, and managing setbacks with grace and self-compassion, we can navigate challenges with confidence and continue to move forward. Remember, setbacks do not define us; it is how we face and overcome them that truly shapes our character and propels us towards success and personal growth.

Finding happiness in the bleakest of situations is not an easy task, but it is possible. It requires cultivating inner strength, shifting perspectives, and finding joy and meaning in small moments. By embracing the present, appreciating beauty, and redefining success and happiness, individuals can navigate war, terminal illness, and other challenging circumstances with greater resilience and a sense of contentment. The human spirit has shown time and again that it is capable of finding happiness amidst even the darkest chapters of life.

Action Time

This is a written action.

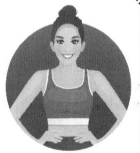

1. Using the space on the following page, write down a challenge that you are facing at the moment.

2. Next, write down three positive things about this challenge. There may be negative things about it as well, but focus on the positive.

3. If you are struggling with this challenge, then come back to these notes and remind yourself of the positives.

My example: I am moving house shortly. Yes, it can be extremely stressful, but the three positive things about moving are: 1. A reduction in a massive mortgage! 2. The chance to buy a new sofa, (I have been wanting to find an excuse for this for years!) and 3. The chance to clear out all the unnecessary and useless rubbish we have accumulated over time.

Exploring habits and addictions

I was a little surprised that addictions were the first two responses I received from my survey – both respondents answered in under a minute to my question online, so it was definitely at the forefront of their minds. In my job, I have to discuss and manage client addictions, and this is a tough subject to bring up. People are very good at playing down or hiding their addictions, and sometimes don't even understand what an addiction is. I decided to write a chapter about this to ensure people understand that it is very common to develop negative habits. Addictions provide temporary happiness, but what damage are they doing in the long term?

Habits

Let's first look at habits. Habits are behaviours that become automatic due to repetition. There are good habits, such as exercising regularly, and bad habits, such as procrastinating. Habits can bring humans temporary happiness because they provide a sense of familiarity and structure to daily life. When we engage in habits, it requires less effort and thought because it has become second nature. This can provide a sense of comfort and ease, leading to a feeling of temporary happiness.

I frequently discuss habit-forming with my clients. Part of my job is to help clients understand their current habits, understand which ones are helpful and which are causing them harm or may be inhibiting progress, and finally to help them build new, helpful habits to reach their goals. A couple of common habits include constantly going to bed too late and eating too late in the day. If these habits are not identified and labelled as such, then discussed as to how they can be altered and a plan formed, then they will remain negative habits that will be detrimental to health and overall happiness.

However, when we engage in bad habits for too long, they can become addictions. Addictions are compulsive behaviours that can interfere with our daily lives. Addictions can range from substance abuse to behavioural addictions, such as gambling or online gaming. Addictions bring temporary happiness by releasing chemicals in our brain that induce pleasure. However, in the long term, these chemicals can become less effective, and more of the substance or behaviour is required to achieve the same level of pleasure. This leads to a cycle of addiction that can have serious long-term consequences.

Addictions

Addiction can have a profound impact on a person's happiness levels. When someone becomes addicted to a substance or behaviour, their brain chemistry undergoes significant changes. Addiction often involves the release of large amounts of dopamine, the neurotransmitter associated with pleasure and reward. However, prolonged and excessive dopamine release due to addiction can lead to a desensitisation of the brain's reward system, resulting in diminished responses to natural rewards and experiences.

As addiction persists, it can adversely affect a person's overall sense of happiness. The compulsive pursuit of an addictive substance or behaviour can become the primary focus of their life, leading to negative consequences such as strained relationships, financial difficulties, and deteriorating physical and mental health. The initial euphoria and pleasure associated with addiction are replaced by feelings of guilt, shame, and dissatisfaction. This can lead to a cycle of addiction, where the individual continues to engage in the addictive behaviour in an attempt to alleviate negative emotions and regain a sense of happiness, only to experience further negative consequences.

Additionally, the excessive release and manipulation of brain chemicals involved in addiction can disrupt the brain's natural reward and pleasure pathways, making it difficult for individuals to experience happiness in other aspects of life. They may become increasingly dependent on the addictive substance or behaviour to experience any semblance of pleasure or happiness, further exacerbating the negative impact on their overall well-being.

When I recently visited the most wonderful museum I have been to in a long time, Body Works in central Amsterdam, one of the sections they looked at was that of human pleasure and how our inner 'reward system' works. They called this 'Pressing the pleasure button.' It is explained below and I found it very helpful in further understanding why we form addictions (and yes, the irony of explaining this whilst in the middle of Amsterdam was not lost on the audience!):

"On an evolutionary level, pleasure is a reward system. It motivates us to repeat things again and again that turn out to be good for survival and reproduction. However, the system has an unhealthy side effect; it is also influential in our susceptibility to addiction.

Humans have learnt to short-circuit the neuronal reward system with cigarettes, alcohol, crack, heroin and other drugs. These drugs activate the dopamine receptors in the brain's pleasure centre – and signalise reward. Because their stimulus is about 10 times more intense than food, these drugs are a powerful motivator. This is why people may become obsessed with them.

Over time, the reward system blunts and needs to be shaken up again with ever larger quantities of the substance to achieve the same effect. As a result, the affected person loses interest in anything else but the next dose, even if his actual survival is at stake." (The Happiness Project)

Overcoming addiction and regaining happiness often require comprehensive treatment and support. By addressing the underlying causes, developing healthy coping mechanisms, and rebuilding a fulfilling life, individuals can gradually restore their happiness levels and establish a more sustainable sense of well-being. But how do we go about practically forming these new habits?

Positive habit forming

Apparently by the end of January over 80% of New Year's resolutions will have fallen by the wayside. It's a sad fact, but we have all been there – best intentions and all that! But why should we form positive habits and what are some tips on how to do this successfully?

As previously discussed, habits are automatic behaviours that our brains develop over time in response to repeated cues and rewards. By creating neural pathways, habits become deeply ingrained patterns of behaviour that require less conscious effort to perform. Research has shown that habits play a critical role in conserving mental energy, allowing our brains to focus on more complex tasks. (Arlinghaus and Johnston, 2019)

Why positive habits matter

Consistency and stability: Habits provide consistency and stability in our lives, creating a sense of order and predictability. By automating repetitive tasks, habits reduce decision fatigue and allow us to navigate our daily routines with ease. This stability promotes a sense of control and reduces stress levels by minimising the need for constant decision-making.

Goal achievement: Many of our aspirations and long-term goals require sustained effort over time. Cultivating positive habits that align with our objectives can significantly increase our chances of success. For instance, if your goal is to become physically fit, forming a habit of regular exercise will help you maintain consistency and progress towards achieving that goal.

Mindset shaping: Habits can influence our mindset and overall mental well-being. By consciously choosing and cultivating habits that align with positive values and goals, we can reshape our thought patterns and develop a more optimistic and growth-oriented mindset. This shift in mindset can enhance our overall happiness and satisfaction with life.

Emotional regulation: Habits have a direct impact on our emotions. Engaging in activities that bring us joy and fulfilment, such as hobbies or spending time with loved ones, can positively affect our emotional well-being. Creating habits around these activities ensures that we regularly experience positive emotions, contributing to an overall sense of happiness.

Creating positive habits

Forming new habits requires a deliberate and systematic approach. By understanding the science of habit formation, we can increase our chances of successfully integrating new habits into our lives. Inspired by *Atomic Habits* by James Clear, below are some hints and tips that could help your New Year's resolution last longer than January.

Small habits can have a large impact on your life:

Begin by focusing on one new habit at a time. Start with a small, achievable action that aligns with your goals. This approach prevents overwhelm and increases the likelihood of success. For example, if your goal is to be able to achieve 100 sit-ups in a row and you are a beginner, it is best to start with doing 10 sit-ups first. Keep adding a couple of sit-ups per day and within a short period of time, you will be quite able to do 100. If you tried to do all 100 on the first day, you would very likely fail. Minor changes each day will lead to bigger results – focus on the trajectory you are heading towards rather than your immediate results.

Building new habits requires a plan of action:

Clearly define the habit you want to form. If you are determined to try to stick to a new habit or goal, create a SMART plan for it. This stands for Specific, Measurable, Achievable, Realistic and Timely. For example, if you simply want to 'get fitter', think of more exact measurements for this: "Within one month, I want to be able to complete a HIIT class, do 10 press ups and walk one mile, and I can practice this on a Monday and a Thursday". In addition, you need to ensure it's realistic; if you have never run before in your life, don't expect to be able to run a marathon within a month! This is covered in more detail in the 'Let's be SMART about this' chapter.

Habits are automated behaviours that we have learnt from experience:

Cues are triggers that prompt the habit, while rewards provide positive reinforcement. By recognising the cues that lead to your desired habits and identifying satisfying rewards, you can reinforce the habit loop and strengthen neural connections. If we try something and it works, we repeat it, especially if it gives us a result we like. For example, if we are trying out a new recipe and it works well and tastes great, we are likely to repeat it. Most households have about 8-10 standard meals that are cooked and repeated. The habit has been formed; we like it, so we repeat it. Habits need a reward, so if we can build positive habits, we will stick to them just as much as the negative ones.

Make habit-forming easier for yourself:

If you leave more obvious cues around your immediate environment to trigger action, this will make forming that new habit much more achievable. For example, if you leave healthy snacks within reach instead of unhealthy snacks, you are much more likely to eat the healthier snacks. If you move your exercise bike into the lounge in front of the TV, you are much more likely to use it than if it's packed up in the spare room. Reduce friction i.e. the effort it takes to do something, and the habit will form much quicker.

Make your habits immediately satisfying:

This is not easy because most goals are not achieved immediately, but if you can attach a positive gratification to it then it will help. For example, using a tracker will help with this as you will see the progress you make each week and month. You could also try putting a £1 coin in the jar every time you go to the gym. This will soon add up to being able to buy funky new trainers!

Summary

The science of habit formation reveals that cultivating positive habits is essential for creating happiness in our lives. By understanding how habits work and leveraging this knowledge, we can consciously shape our behaviours and mindset to support our aspirations and well-being. Remember, happiness is not a destination but a journey, and forming habits that align with our values and goals can help us navigate that journey with greater satisfaction and fulfilment.

It is important to acknowledge the temporary happiness provided by habits and addictions, but also to recognise the long-term consequences. Good habits can lead to a structured and comfortable daily routine, while bad habits can develop into addictions that harm your physical and mental health. It's important to seek help if struggling with addiction and to work towards developing good habits that benefit overall well-being.

Action Time

This is a written action.

1. Using the space underneath, write down two good habits you would like to have in your life, but don't currently at the moment.

2. Using the advice in this chapter, see if you can manage to do one of them for at least a month.

My example: I would like to form the habit of practicing yoga at least twice per week, even if it's only 20 minutes per session.

1B – HAPPINESS SURVEY

We are family

Sharing time with family and friends was the most popular answer of my survey of 'What makes you happy?'. Of all the creatures on earth, humans are unique in their need and desire to interact and form communities. Our social bonds provide us with a sense of belonging and connection that is essential to our physical and emotional well-being. In this chapter, we will delve into the science behind why we like to be with family and friends, and explore the importance of community.

The science of social bonding

From an evolutionary perspective, the need for social bonds can be traced back to our primate ancestors. These primates formed groups to protect themselves from predators and to increase their chances of finding food. In humans, these basic needs have evolved into a more complex set of social and emotional needs.

Studies have shown that social bonding triggers the release of certain hormones, such as oxytocin and endorphins. There is a particularly interesting study by the Karolinska Institute in Stockholm, suggesting that if oxytocin is released into our systems daily for five days, this can decrease blood pressure, decrease stress hormone levels (cortisol), and promote faster healing of wounds. (Uvnas-Moberg et al, 2014)

Oxytocin is often referred to as the 'love hormone' because it is released during activities such as breastfeeding, hugging, and sex. It promotes feelings of trust, empathy, and bonding. Endorphins, on the other hand, are responsible for providing a sense of pleasure and pain relief – this is often felt when finishing a run or a good weightlifting session in the gym.

The importance of community

Humans are social animals, and our connections to others play a vital role in maintaining our physical and mental health. Research has shown that individuals who have strong social ties live longer, are less likely to develop chronic diseases, and have better mental health outcomes.

"People in neighbourhoods with higher levels of social cohesion experience lower rates of mental health problems than those in neighbourhoods with lower cohesion, independent of how deprived or affluent a neighbourhood is." (mentalhealth.org.uk)

One study in the Journal of the American Geriatrics Society found that individuals who reported having a lower number of social connections were also much more likely to develop dementia – a 27% increased chance. (Huang et al, 2023)

Another study, analysing the findings of 90 separate studies involving 2,205,199 people, found that social isolation was associated with a higher risk of mortality. The connections we form with others can provide us with a sense of purpose and meaning in life.

"The large meta-analysis found that being socially isolated was associated with a 26% increase in the risk of all-cause death compared to people who were not socially isolated. The effect of loneliness was slightly less but still concerning: the chance of death for people experiencing prolonged loneliness was 14% higher than for people who were not lonely." (Robby Berman, 2023)

Family bonds

The importance of family in fostering happiness cannot be overstated. Family bonds are the foundation of social ties, and our connections with family members can have a profound impact on our lives.

Firstly, the family usually serves as a source of unconditional love and acceptance. In a world that can be harsh and judgemental, knowing that there are loved ones who accept us for who we are brings immense comfort and happiness. Family members offer a safe space where we can be vulnerable, express our true selves, and receive love and reassurance without judgement. This unwavering support creates a sense of emotional security, significantly enhancing our overall happiness.

Moreover, the family provides a support network during both times of joy and times of adversity. When we achieve a personal milestone or celebrate a success (the A-level and GCSE results have been announced as I am writing this – lots of family celebrations happening this weekend!), sharing these moments with family members amplifies our happiness. Their genuine excitement and pride validate our accomplishments and reinforce our sense of self-worth.

During challenging times, such as facing illness or going through difficult life transitions, family members often rally together to provide emotional, financial, and practical support. Knowing that we can lean on our family in times of need provides a sense of comfort and relief, easing the burden and helping us navigate the challenges with greater resilience and optimism.

Furthermore, family offers us a sense of belonging and connection. Human beings are social creatures, and having a loving family helps satisfy our innate need for social interaction and belongingness. Sharing experiences, traditions, and values with our family members fosters a strong sense of identity and roots that contribute to our overall happiness.

Research has also shown that family members who regularly spend time with one another have lower levels of stress and greater emotional resilience.

"Stress process theory suggests that the positive and negative aspects of relationships can have a large impact on the well-being of individuals. Family relationships provide resources that can help an individual cope with stress, engage in healthier behaviors, and enhance self-esteem, leading to higher well-being." (Thomas et al, 2017)

Family also plays a crucial role in shaping our personal development. As we grow, our interactions with family members help us acquire important skills, values, and beliefs. Through their guidance, encouragement, and example, family members help us develop a solid moral compass, cultivate empathy, and navigate through life's complexities. These qualities contribute not only to our personal growth, but also to our ability to build and maintain healthy relationships with others, further enhancing our happiness.

One study found that children who have a strong attachment to their parents are more likely to have positive relationships with their friends and are less likely to engage in risky behaviours such as drug use and delinquency. In addition, strong family bonds can provide a buffer against the stresses and challenges of daily life.

"According to attachment theory, children's early experiences with their primary caregivers, in terms of protection and security, are the basis for socio-emotional development and for the establishment of close relationships throughout their lives. During adolescence, friends and peers become a primary developmental environment, and thereby establishing quality bonds with peers will foster good psychological adjustment." (Delgado et al, 2018)

Friendship

Friendship is another important aspect of social bonding that can have a significant impact on our lives. Friendships hold a significant role in our pursuit of happiness and overall well-being. Genuine friendships provide us with emotional support, companionship, and a sense of belonging, filling our lives with joy and fulfilment. They say you can't choose your family, but you can choose your friends!

One of the key aspects of friendships is the emotional support they offer. True friends are those who genuinely care about our well-being and are there to listen, offer advice, and provide comfort when we face hardships. Having someone who understands and empathises with our struggles can be immensely comforting and uplifting. The emotional bond formed through friendship acts as a buffer against stress, anxiety, and loneliness, promoting better mental health and contributing to our happiness.

Friendships also serve as a vital source of companionship and shared experiences. Engaging in activities, hobbies, or simply spending quality time with friends brings joy, laughter, and a sense of belonging. The shared moments of laughter, celebration, and even simply everyday interactions create memories that make life more meaningful and enjoyable. Having friends to share our joys and sorrows with, provides a sense of connection and deepens our appreciation for life, ultimately contributing to our happiness.

Before writing this part of the chapter, I had been on a lovely walk with my dog and a friend. We both enjoy walking and chatting, as this activity brings us closer together. After the walk, we felt relaxed and happy that we had chatted about things we wanted to share or were worried about. In addition, the dog had a very long walk and is very happily asleep next to me! Wins all round!

Friendships also provide us with a diverse and unique support system beyond our immediate family. While family bonds are foundational, friendships offer a different perspective and provide alternative sources of support. Friends often challenge us, help us grow, and introduce us to new ideas, experiences, and opportunities. In times of personal growth or decision-making, trusted friends can offer guidance, feedback, and different viewpoints that broaden our horizons and contribute to personal development.

Research has shown that individuals who have close friendships are happier and have better mental health outcomes – possibly even more important for your health than exercise. One study found that having social support from friends can help mitigate the negative effects of stress on mental health.

"A landmark study by Holt-Lunstad et al at Brigham Young University conducted a meta-analysis and found that having a few close friends was more important for health outcomes (think: high blood pressure, heart disease, depression, cancer) than diet or exercise habits." (Holt-Lunstad et al, 2015)

Friendships also play a crucial role in shaping our identity and self-esteem. Friends' acceptance and appreciation for who we are allow us to feel valued and loved for our individuality. Building strong and meaningful friendships can contribute to higher self-esteem, as positive feedback and affirmation from friends reaffirm our worth. Having friends who genuinely support and believe in us can boost our confidence and give us the courage to pursue our dreams and aspirations, leading to greater happiness and personal success.

Summary

The science behind why we like to be with family and friends has shown that social connections are vital to our physical and emotional well-being. Strong social bonds can provide us with a sense of purpose and meaning in life, help us cope with the stresses of daily life, and contribute to a longer and healthier life. So, whether it's spending time with loved ones or cultivating new friendships, taking the time to connect with others is an essential part of a healthy and happier life.

Action time

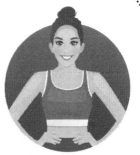

This is a practical action.

1. In your local community, research the fun events that are available throughout the year.

2. Look at local newspapers/magazines, websites, Facebook groups and noticeboards where details can be found.

3. Pick one, go along with family and friends, and see what you think.

4. Are you surprised there is so much? (and a lot of it for free!) I thought so!

My example: I am planning on going to my local Christmas market at the beginning of December with the family. A great way to start the festive cheer!

Love actually, is...

"If you look for it, I've got a sneaky feeling you'll find that love, actually, is all around."

Love Actually – film, directed by Richard Curtis

I can't write a book about happiness without touching on the subject of love. Having recently listened to Simon Sinek's brilliant podcast interview of Richard Curtis, it inspired me; the topic of 'lurvvvvve' and the happiness and joy this can bring. I say 'can', because it also brings an exposure to vulnerability and potential heartache.

I am lucky enough to remember the last time I fell in love and saying 'I feel love-sick' – there is definitely some truth to this. It is the strangest combination of intense, complete and utter elation combined with an almost physical 'ache' that you are not with each other every moment of the day when you both want to be. This honeymoon period settles down, of course, but what follows should be calm, comfort, contentment, and a more sustainable happiness.

From a scientific perspective, what happens in our bodies to produce this feeling of love, creating an intense happiness, and why does this feeling change over time? Scientific research has unravelled many mysteries, shedding light on the physiological and psychological processes that initiate and sustain our feelings of love.

The biological dance of love

Our emotional experience of love is tightly intertwined with a symphony of biological processes. At the core of this dance lies the brain, where the release of neurotransmitters and hormones orchestrates our amorous emotions.

Neuronal fireworks: When we fall in love, the brain's pleasure centres, such as the ventral tegmental area, are activated, leading to the release of neurotransmitters like dopamine, oxytocin, and serotonin. Dopamine, often referred to as the 'pleasure molecule', is responsible for the elation and euphoria experienced during the initial stages of love. It reinforces the reward circuitry of the brain, creating an addiction-like response to the presence of the beloved.

The oxytocin connection: Oxytocin, popularly known as the 'love hormone', is released in abundance during moments of intimacy, physical touch, and bonding activities between individuals. It fosters feelings of trust, connection, and emotional bonding. Oxytocin also plays a significant role in promoting empathy and socialisation, making it a crucial element in the formation and maintenance of long-term relationships.

Serotonin setting: Serotonin, another neurotransmitter, is responsible for regulating mood, social behaviour, and well-being. It acts as a stabiliser during the initial stage of romantic attachment, promoting feelings of contentment and happiness. However, as love transitions from an intense infatuation stage to a more stable relationship, serotonin levels can plateau or decrease, leading to a decrease in romantic intensity and the infamous honeymoon period coming to an end.

Why love changes over time

Despite the initial intensity of romantic love, no feeling can escape change. Sometimes this is difficult to come to terms with, but it is fruitless fighting it. Over time, the flames of passion fluctuate, leading to different dynamics within relationships. Several factors contribute to why love changes:

Biological adaptation: Our biological systems are designed to adapt to new experiences, including love. As we get used to the presence of a romantic partner, our brain chemistry undergoes alterations, reducing the extent of the dopamine-induced pleasure response. This adaptation is crucial for long-term bonding, as it enables us to focus on other aspects of the relationship, such as building trust, shared interests, and deeper emotional connections.

Familiarity and routine: The initial stages of love are filled with novelty and excitement. However, human beings tend to seek stability and routine, which can inadvertently diminish the initial spark. Familiarity can bring comfort, but it can also lead to a decrease in the frequency of surprise or novelty, impacting the intensity of love over time.

Emotional intimacy vs. passionate love: Love takes on different forms as it evolves. While the fiery passion may decrease, emotional intimacy and attachment tend to grow stronger in long-term relationships. The brain shifts its focus from infatuation to maintaining a deeper emotional connection, where oxytocin plays a vital role. Emotional intimacy fosters a sense of security, trust, and the ability to weather the challenges that life may bring.

However, it also made me think about potential differences between men and women when it comes to experiencing love. Research suggests that there are both similarities and subtle differences in how men and women experience love due to biological and societal factors. It's important to note that these findings are generalisations and may not hold true for every individual.

Biological Factors

Biologically, there are some distinctions in the ways men and women experience love. I was, however, a little surprised about results from this particular study:

A study by Harrison and Shortall (2011) found that *"men tend to fall in love faster than women. Contrary to popular belief that women are the first to be more expressive in a relationship, the study showed that men are more likely to say 'I love you' first."*

Brain function: Studies using brain imaging techniques have revealed that men and women tend to activate different areas of the brain during emotional experiences. Women often show more activity in brain regions associated with emotional processing, empathy, and bonding, such as the limbic system and prefrontal cortex. Men, on the other hand, may exhibit increased activation in areas related to reward and pleasure, like the amygdala and nucleus accumbens. (Hai-Jiang Li et al, 2014)

Hormonal influences: Hormones, such as oestrogen and testosterone, also play a role in shaping emotional experiences. Research indicates that oestrogen enhances the effects of oxytocin, which is linked to feelings of bonding and connection. Testosterone, more prevalent in men, can influence desires for novelty, competition, and sexual attraction, potentially contributing to variations in love experiences. (van Anders et al, 2015)

Societal factors

In addition to biological factors, societal influences also contribute to differences in how men and women experience love.

Cultural expectations: Societal norms and expectations often shape individuals' behaviours and expressions of love. For instance, women may be socialised to emphasise emotional intimacy and promote relationship satisfaction, while men may be encouraged to focus on passion, sexual desire, and providing for their partners. These social constructs can influence the way each gender perceives and expresses love.

Relationship priorities: Research suggests that men and women may prioritise different aspects of love in relationships. Women may place greater value on emotional security, communication, and connection, while men may prioritise physical intimacy and sexual satisfaction. These variations can affect the way love is experienced and expressed between the genders.

I read an interesting article from the Relationship Institute, called *Differences Between Men and Women*, that delved into relationship priorities for men and women and there were some useful adjectives that were explored. Apparently, women need to receive care, understanding, respect, devotion, validation, and reassurance, and are motivated when they are made to feel special or cherished. However, men need to receive trust, acceptance, appreciation, admiration, approval, and encouragement. Discussing this with my husband who happened to be next to me when I was reading this, he suggested that everyone's needs are different, but his priorities revolved around beer, sport, and his mobile phone! I left the conversation there... !

After having a more productive conversation with a younger, male (heterosexual) friend of mine who is currently on the dating scene, he did have an opposite opinion to the above though. When going out to find a potential person to date, the women tend to be the 'peacock' – looking beautiful and amazing to attract a partner. His view was that men need to trust the lady they are dating to fend off other potential men who might be looking at their attractiveness. Women want respect from the man they have chosen to date so that they don't go off looking for another 'peacock'.

Summary

Love is not solely a product of emotional experience, but also a complex interplay of biological processes within our bodies. Dopamine, oxytocin, serotonin, and other chemicals shape our romantic relationships from the initial exhilaration to the evolution towards deeper emotional connections. Love experiences are also influenced by a myriad of factors including personal history, cultural backgrounds, individual preferences, and subtle differences in the way males and females experience love. Understanding the biology and societal factors of love can help us appreciate its nuances, navigate its changes, and cherish the transformative power and deep happiness it can hold in our lives.

Action Time

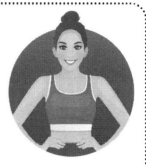

This is a written action.

1. Think about a person you have in your life that you love and, using the space on the following page, write down five reasons why you love them.

2. Then text or WhatsApp this person, telling them that you love them and the reasons why. It's always amazing to hear and it will make their day!

My example: I don't tell my husband I love him enough, so I think having it in print for the rest of time is a pretty good gesture !!☺

-   He is always there for me, in whatever mood or state I am in.

-   He is very practical and organised and brings this skill to organising our household.

-   He has helped to produce two very cute kids – they look just like him!

-   He is a very good listener – I am a very good talker!

-   He is very resourceful and has always provided for us as a family as to whatever is needed.

Thank you, Sam. My rock.

Why do pets have such a positive impact on our lives?

This was another very popular answer in my survey. I was a little surprised at how high up this scored, but being the owner of little Teddy the Cavapoo, who is an integral part of our family and definitely my favourite child (!), I get it! He is sitting right next to me now as I type. Bless him!

Pets have been a part of human society for thousands of years and have been valued as companions, protectors, and even spiritual entities. Over time, the benefits of pet ownership have become increasingly recognised and studied by researchers. Today, it is widely accepted that pets have a positive impact on our lives in many ways. COVID exacerbated pet ownership as well:

"While the estimated population of dogs, cats and rabbits remain similar to pre-pandemic levels, 24% of all owners acquired their pet in the last two years, equating to 5.4 million pets acquired since the start of the pandemic in March 2020." (PDSA Paw Report, 2022)

Here are a few suggestions as to why pets make such great companions:

Reduce stress and anxiety

One of the most significant benefits of having a pet is the calming effect they can have on our emotions. Research has shown that pets, particularly dogs, can decrease blood pressure and lower levels of stress hormones like cortisol. Pets can also provide a sense of comfort and security, especially for those who live alone or have experienced trauma.

An article from *News In Health*, 'The Power of Pets', looked at specific studies where animals were brought in to help people: *"Dogs are very present. If someone is struggling with something, they know how to sit there and be loving... Their attention is focused on the person all the time."* (2018)

Improve mental health

It's not simply our physical health that benefits from pet ownership. Studies have also shown that pets can improve our mental health as well. For instance, pets can increase feelings of happiness and reduce symptoms of depression. The emotional support and companionship pets provide can even help people with conditions like PTSD and social anxiety disorder. The reason we got our little Cavapoo, Teddy, was to try to help with our son Charlie's ADHD and autism. Although we all adore our dog, Charlie and Teddy have an extra special bond and the dog seems to know when Charlie needs support and when he doesn't. Charlie finds it particularly comforting to stroke the top of Teddy's head (he has a very soft head!) in a repetitive motion that calms Charlie and that Teddy enjoys as well.

One of the corporate clients I work with recently introduced a very interesting, different monthly social team activity that gets voted by the staff. A few months ago they decided to stray away from the usual pub visits (to be fair, they usually go down well!) and asked a specialist company called Paws in Work (www.pawsinwork.com) to bring in a litter of puppies for staff to cuddle and play with instead. It was ridiculously cute and went down so well with the team that they have added it to their social calendar every quarter! Afterwards, staff reported they felt calmer, happier, and much more positive towards their company and the teammates with whom they shared the experience.

Encourage exercise

When it comes to taking care of dogs, exercise is important. Dogs need to go for a walk every day, come rain or shine! This means that dog owners are more likely to keep up their steps as well, going for walks or playing 'fetch' with their furry friends. Maintaining an active lifestyle is not only good for physical health, it can also help boost your mood and reduce stress.

Reduce loneliness and increase social interaction

Pets can be an excellent social catalyst, helping their owners meet others who share a common bond. Whether it's at the park, pet shop, or a community event, pet owners have the opportunity to bond over their love of animals. I can't go five minutes down the road without someone stopping me to ask if they can pet Teddy, and then naturally having a chat to me as well. This can help to reduce feelings of loneliness and increase social interaction, which is important for our mental and emotional well-being.

The Guardian agrees and stated in an article in March 2020 that dogs in particular have a 'magical' effect on the positivity of our mental health: *"The importance of social recognition is increasingly acknowledged for the role it plays in helping us form networks. We now understand that healthy social bonds can play a key role in mental health; without them, we become lonely, depressed and physically unwell. And pets, it seems, can fulfil that role."*

Provide a sense of purpose

Lastly, pets can provide a sense of purpose and responsibility. Caring for a pet requires daily attention and routine, which can help increase our sense of structure and meaning in life. Knowing that your pet relies on you for their needs can also give you a sense of purpose and fulfilment.

Summary

Overall, pets have a positive impact on our lives in many ways. Whether you're a dog person, cat person, or prefer something more exotic, having a pet can bring lots of happiness, companionship, and positivity to our daily lives. Of course, they need a level of looking after and this comes with responsibility, energy, and time, but the benefits very much outweigh the effort.

Action Time

This is a practical action.

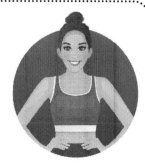

1. Depending on where (or if) you work, go and have a chat with HR and see if dogs are allowed in your office.

2. If you have a dog, and HR agree, bring your dog to work one day. It helps to elevate everyone's mood and you will be pleasantly surprised how many people want to come and pet the dog and have a chat with you at the same time. Dogs soften even the hardest of co-workers!

3. If you don't have a dog, see if one of your colleagues is allowed to bring their dog into the office.

My example: I bring Teddy to work frequently (little therapy dog!) and I'm sure people come to the gym to see him, rather than me!

Our chosen hobbies

I have definitely had a number of hobbies in my life – some of them have come and gone as I realise that I am absolutely hopeless at them and should perhaps move on (tennis springs to mind!), and others have formed a large part of my life for years (painting, sewing, baking, interior design, and gymnastics). My hobbies may alter but I would be lost without having any.

In the hustle and bustle of our busy lives, it's essential to find time for ourselves and engage in activities that bring us joy, which may not be that easy. This is where the significance of having hobbies lies. Hobbies not only serve as a means of relaxation and escape from the daily grind but also provide numerous benefits that positively impact our overall happiness and well-being. Not surprisingly, enjoying hobbies featured highly in my happiness survey. In this chapter, we explore the importance of having hobbies and how they enhance our happiness.

A source of emotional fulfilment

Hobbies serve as an outlet for our creativity and self-expression, allowing us to engage in activities that bring us joy and fulfilment. Whether it's painting, writing, playing a musical instrument, or gardening, hobbies enable us to tap into our passions, providing a sense of purpose and contentment. Engaging in activities that align with our interests allows us to experience positive emotions, leading to increased happiness and satisfaction in life.

Stress relief and mental well-being

The demands of our modern lives can often leave us feeling overwhelmed and stressed. Hobbies offer a much-needed break from our daily responsibilities and provide a sense of relaxation and calmness. Immersing ourselves in a favourite pastime, such as practising yoga, going for a run, or engaging in a hobby that utilises our hands like knitting or woodworking, can help reduce stress levels and promote mental well-being. Hobbies provide an escape from our worries and serve as a healthy coping mechanism for dealing with life's challenges.

Boosting self-confidence and self-esteem

Pursuing hobbies allows us to acquire new skills and improve existing ones. As we dedicate time and effort to mastering our hobbies, we experience a sense of accomplishment and increased self-confidence. Whether it's learning a new language, cooking a gourmet meal, or playing a sport, hobbies give us opportunities to set goals, track progress, and celebrate our achievements. This, in turn, improves our self-esteem and overall happiness.

Building social connections and a sense of belonging

Hobbies often bring people together, fostering a sense of community and belonging. Engaging in group activities or joining clubs and organisations related to our hobbies provides opportunities to meet like-minded individuals who share similar interests. These social connections not only provide a support network, but also contribute to a sense of belonging, ultimately boosting our happiness and overall well-being. Whether it's attending book clubs, joining sports leagues, or participating in community art projects, hobbies offer avenues for building meaningful relationships.

"Countless studies have found that social connection is a key component of happiness and a meaningful life, and hobbies have the potential to create precious new ties." (Jamie Kurtz, 2015)

As an example, my eldest son, Charlie, has transformed from a bored, disruptive and holding too much unchannelled energy teenager, into a sports champion with purpose, focus, and a true sense of belonging. From school drop-out to revered by the school for being a high achiever – not academically, but just by using his hobby to create a career and true happiness for himself. *"When I am karting it makes me feel like I'm invincible; I love the adrenaline, the speed, the power of the kart, and who I race against – everyone there is like me, we love it!"*

I would also like to reference another mini-man that has a similar hobby but for very different reasons. My youngest son, Harry, is a remote control (RC) car racer – not quite as dangerous as being in the car, of course, but they can still crash and catch fire! He absolutely loves his hobby, but not for the speed or chemical rush but to understand the mechanics of the car and fiddle about with incrementally improving the car's performance. He is just so happy when he has a race weekend – even if he doesn't win, it's the sense of belonging he enjoys the most.

Summary

Hobbies play a vital role in enhancing our happiness and well-being. They provide us with emotional fulfilment, act as a stress reliever, boost our self-confidence, and help us build social connections. By dedicating time to the activities we love, we cultivate a greater sense of joy, purpose, and contentment in our lives. Therefore, it's essential to prioritise hobbies and make time for them amidst our busy schedules. So, go ahead, pursue that passion you've been putting off, and experience the transformative power of hobbies.

Action Time

This is a written action.

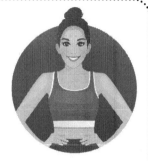

1. Using the space below, write down a hobby that you would like to give a try, either on your own or with a friend/partner/child. Be creative – there are hundreds of options out there!

2. Research where you could do this hobby locally. Is it at a club? Or at your house if you have room?

My examples: Jewellery making, darts, aerial yoga, baking, stamp collecting, and unicycle riding!

Music for the soul

"When a beautiful piece of music moves us to tears or sends chills down our back, the areas that light up in the brain include those activated when we indulge in our greatest pleasures. Our heart rate and respiration change. Blood flows increase in those parts of the brain associated with reward, motivation and arousal." (The Happiness Project)

Music, with its harmonious melodies and captivating rhythms, has the remarkable ability to evoke deep emotional experiences within us. Whether it's a joyful tune that makes us want to dance, or a soothing melody that lulls us into a relaxed state, music has been celebrated throughout history for its profound impact on our well-being. Most people have experienced hearing a tune again that reminds them of a time in their life or a certain person – I love it when this happens! In this chapter, we explore the positive benefits of music, and how it can provide us with strong feelings of happiness at any given moment in our lives.

The therapeutic effects of music

Music has long been recognised as a powerful therapeutic tool that can positively impact our mental and physical health. An article in VerywellMind.com details how listening to music can reduce stress and anxiety by promoting the release of endorphins, which are natural feel-good chemicals in our brains. When we listen to music we enjoy, our bodies respond by lowering levels of cortisol, the stress hormone, thereby creating a sense of relaxation and calm.

"With alterations in brainwaves comes changes in other bodily functions. Those governed by the autonomic nervous system, such as breathing and heart rate can also be altered by the changes music can bring. This can mean slower breathing, slower heart rate and an activation of the relaxation response." (Scott, 2020)

In addition to reducing stress, music has the ability to enhance our mood and increase happiness. Certain songs or genres can evoke feelings of joy, nostalgia, or excitement, transporting us to a state of euphoria. We often find ourselves uplifted and rejuvenated after a session of listening to our favourite tunes.

Earlier this year, I went to Ushuaia, one of the biggest and most impressive clubs in Ibiza. The DJ Calvin Harris was headlining. Being in a club with 5,000 other people all soaking up every moment of that experience is beyond words – I cannot tell you how powerful and positive this felt! Before writing this chapter, I have just been dancing around the kitchen with my sister listening to Calvin Harris and remembering when we were at Ushuaia – all it took was a song and we were transported back there, so happy and loving life!

The connection between music and the brain

I have often wondered why certain songs have the power to evoke emotion or trigger memories. It lies in the way our brains process music. When we listen to music, multiple areas of our brain become activated, including those responsible for emotion, memory, and motivation.

Neurological studies have shown that music stimulates the release of dopamine, a neurotransmitter associated with pleasure and reward. This explains why music can generate such strong emotions and feelings of happiness. Additionally, when we listen to a familiar song, it can trigger memories, taking us back to specific moments in our lives that were associated with that particular piece of music. This link between music and memory is a profound phenomenon, allowing us to relive experiences and emotions simply through the power of sound.

"Music has (also) been found to bring many other benefits, such as lowering blood pressure, boost immunity, ease muscle tension and

more. With so many benefits and such profound physical effects, it's no surprise that so many are seeing music as an important tool to help the body in staying, or becoming, healthy." (Scott, 2020)

Creating personal playlists for relaxation

One of the beautiful aspects of music is its wide variety, catering to individual preferences and moods. Creating personalised playlists can be a valuable tool for relaxation. Experiment with different genres, styles, and tempos to curate a collection of songs that resonate with you. I experiment with this frequently in the gym; blast out some 80s power ballads and you will find that people move much faster and lift heavier weights! Play some calm, easy-listening tunes and people will opt to stretch for a little longer on the mats!

For relaxation and unwinding, consider incorporating slow-tempo melodies, gentle instrumentals, or ambient soundscapes into your playlist. These types of music have the power to slow down your breathing and heart rate, promoting a state of deep relaxation. Experiment with different genres such as classical, jazz, or nature-inspired compositions to find what works best for you.

Integrating music into daily life

Incorporating music into your daily routine can significantly enhance your happiness and well-being. Start your day on a positive note by playing uplifting tunes while getting ready in the morning. I usually have the radio on in the car on my way to work – even very early in the morning, a few pop tunes will prep me for my long day of personal training sessions. During breaks, take a moment to listen to a favourite song and allow yourself to be fully immersed in the experience, even if it is for one song.

I couldn't write a chapter about music without referencing my sister's favourite, meaningful song *Everybody's Free (to wear sunscreen)* by Baz Luhrmann. However, the words themselves were written by a columnist for the Chicago Tribune, Mary Schmich, in 1997. She presents this as the commencement of a speech she would give if ever asked (I hope she was asked, it would have been fabulous!!). It is a song about getting older and what you would say to your younger self. The key take-outs are hidden throughout the song: Wear sunscreen, enjoy your youth, try not to worry too much, floss, don't be jealous of others, stretch, take calcium for your joints, dance, travel, and respect your elders. I think the advice here is certainly worth noting and will definitely make you a happier person.

I think the most appropriate section of the song for me is: *"Enjoy your body, use it every way you can. Don't be afraid of it or what other people think of it. It's the greatest instrument you'll ever own."*

Summary

Using the power of music to relax and bring happiness into our lives cannot be overstated. Its therapeutic effects on our mind and body are incredible, and we have the opportunity to harness this power for our own well-being quite easily. By deliberately incorporating music into our daily routines and creating personal playlists, we can unlock a strong level of happiness within ourselves. So, put on your favourite song, close your eyes, and let the magic of music wash over you, bringing relaxation and joy to your soul.

Action Time

This is a written action.

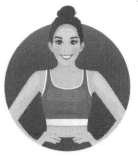

1. Using the space on the following page, list some of your favourite songs/pieces of music.

2. Now write down what kind of mood each piece brings and what emotions each of them evokes for you.

3. Now write down if these songs remind you of a certain person, place, or activity.

My example:

Song 1 – *Set You Free* by N-Trance. An absolute club classic! Every time I hear this upbeat dance tune, it puts me in a good mood, heightens my energy levels, and reminds me of one of my oldest friends, Natasha, and how back in the day, when we were young, getting into clubs when we weren't old enough and dancing the night away.

Song 2 – *Everywhere* by Fleetwood Mac, an 80s classic! When I hear this song, it reminds me of one of my best friends, Chris. It's also one of his favourite songs. It provokes a calm and tranquil happiness in me and I feel I can just float away from my worries.

Material girl

"In our modern world, we surround ourselves with lots of material possessions. But they haven't made us any happier. Rather, happiness is influenced by our choices – our inner attitudes, how we approach our relationships, our personal values and our sense of purpose." (The Happiness Project)

We all want to live a happy life, but we often mistakenly believe that material possessions or more money will bring us that happiness. This, however, is not always the case; do possessions and more cash make us truly happy?

First, it's important to recognise that there's no single answer to this question. After all, what brings one person happiness might not bring another person happiness. However, research suggests that material possessions and pots of cash alone aren't enough to lead to deep and lasting happiness.

Material possessions are usually fleeting. We might get a temporary boost in happiness from buying a new car or a fashionable piece of clothing, but that happiness is likely to fade over time. Once the novelty and excitement die down, we're often left searching for the next thing that will make us happy. (Does this mean that my second book needs to be started shortly?!) This constant cycle of acquisition can lead to stress, anxiety and, ultimately, dissatisfaction.

I also wondered about financial wealth and the many material choices we could make. If we are given more, does this help us and make us happier? It would be logical to assume that the more choices we have, the better. But research tells us this is surprisingly not necessarily the case. The 'chocolate test' was developed by Sheena S Iyengar from Columbia University and Mark R Lepper from Stanford University, in January 2000. (I wish I had been part of this!!)

"Students were invited to participate in a study where they would sample chocolates to determine how satisfied they were with their choices and likelihood to purchase as a result of their sampling. Group A was given a single piece of chocolate, Group B was asked to select one piece out of six offerings. Group C was asked to choose one piece out of thirty different chocolates.

The results showed that less is sometimes more. Those who could choose one chocolate out of thirty were unhappier with their choice than those who could choose out of six different sorts. However, those who were least satisfied were those individuals who had no choice at all."

If we have learnt anything from watching chef Gordon Ramsey's *Kitchen Nightmares* TV show, it's that if a restaurant menu is very long, there are too many choices for people and they don't like it! The French have a very fitting saying: 'embarras de choix'. Cut the menu right down as customers much prefer just a few options – in addition, the quality and efficiency of what comes out of the kitchen is vastly improved as well.

Additionally, there's a phenomenon known as the hedonic treadmill. This is the idea that we adapt to changes in our lives very quickly – including changes in our material possessions. Something that brings us immense happiness and satisfaction at first will soon become the new normal, and we'll start to crave even more. If you have children, you will see them experience this frequently!

On the other hand, experiences tend to bring more lasting happiness than material possessions. Experiences such as travelling, attending an event that we've been looking forward to, or spending quality time with our loved ones, can create memories and positive emotions that stay with us for a long time. These experiences also tend to be richer and more meaningful than simply buying something new.

It's all about the money, money, money!

In today's society, we are conditioned to believe that financial success is the key to happiness. We are constantly bombarded with messages that suggest that owning bigger cars, larger houses, and having more money will automatically make us happy. However, the question remains: Does financial success bring true happiness?

Studies have shown that money does play a role in an individual's happiness, but only to a certain extent. According to a 2010 Princeton study, by Angus Deaton and Daniel Kahneman, your happiness level increases as your income rises, but once you reach an income of $75,000 per year (circa £50,000), the impact of money on your happiness begins to decrease. In other words, money can only buy happiness up to a certain point. However, *The Guardian* published an article in 2023, suggesting that the tipping point in the UK is now nearer the £83,000 mark (depending on your geographical area).

There are several reasons why big financial success may not bring happiness. First, the quest for money can often lead to high levels of stress and anxiety. Individuals who are focused solely on accumulating wealth may neglect other areas of their lives, such as spending quality time with family and friends, pursuing hobbies and passions, or engaging in meaningful activities that bring them joy. A number of my very good friends and clients are prime examples of this; they are very successful in their work life and are extremely high-earning individuals, but are constantly experiencing dangerously high stress levels, and have problems with family life and relationships because they are always working – they would not describe themselves as 'happy and content' at all.

Second, having more money can lead to feelings of isolation and disconnection from others. Wealthy individuals may struggle to form meaningful relationships because they worry about others' intentions and are concerned about being taken advantage of for what they have. This can cause a sense of loneliness, which can lead to poor mental health.

Third, the pursuit of wealth can be a never-ending cycle. There will always be a desire for more, newer, and better things. No matter how much money we have, there will always be someone who has more, and the temptation to keep up and acquire more can be overwhelming.

On the flip side, those who live simple or modest lives in terms of money tend to experience more freedom, fulfilment, and inner peace in life. This may be because they focus on the things that truly matter in life, like building meaningful relationships, pursuing their passions, learning new things, and contributing to society in another way.

Is there a middle ground perhaps? Can you earn enough to pursue your dreams and achieve what you would like to, but not be constantly worrying about your financial situation, or constant pressure from work to over-perform due to fear of getting fired? There are thousands of self-help books out there that promise to help you earn more by eventually doing less.

A favourite of mine is *The 4-Hour Work Week* by Timothy Ferris. He describes how to break away from the slavery of the nine-to-five office job to create a source of continuous and passive income that requires minimal input from you each week, once set up. Another favourite is *Your Money or Your Life* by Vicki Robin and Joe Dominguez, which discusses nine steps to taking control of your finances so you feel able to enjoy life rather than living to work.

Finally, research suggests that having strong social connections and a sense of purpose in life are two of the biggest predictors of happiness. It's hard to build strong connections or a sense of purpose by simply buying more things. These things require time and effort to build, but the effort we put into building them tends to pay off in the form of greater long-term happiness.

Summary

While material possessions can provide a temporary boost in happiness, they're not the key to lasting happiness. True happiness comes from experiences, strong relationships, and a sense of purpose in life. Similarly, while money can bring temporary happiness and security, it may not be the key to long-term happiness and well-being. Simply having more money does not guarantee happiness, and often, the quest for financial success can lead to more stress, anxiety, and disconnection from those around us. Instead of focusing solely on accumulating wealth and possessions, it may be more beneficial to focus on building a fulfilling and meaningful life, incorporating financial stability into the larger picture, and striking a balance between the two. Remember, true happiness ultimately comes from within, not from external sources like money.

> *"It's not how much we have, but how much we enjoy,*
> *that makes happiness."*

Charles Spurgeon (1834 – 1892)
British Baptist Preacher

Action Time

This is a written action.

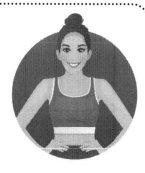

1. Using the space below, write down one activity you would like to do or try for the first time that doesn't cost you any money.

2. Schedule this activity in your diary.

3. After you have completed the activity, note down how you feel. You are likely to find that you had just as much fun (possibly even more!) than if you had done something expensive.

My example: There are hundreds of activities that are free to visit or take part in including; parks, museums, walks, libraries, and local community events. In my diary I have scheduled a bike ride along part of the Thames Path, where I will stop for a little picnic and watch the world go by.

Booked it. Packed it. F * *cked off...

At the time of writing this, I am definitely not on holiday or in my happy place! Although it's July in the UK, it's tipping down with rain and it's unseasonably cold! My mood is definitely affected, and I am very much wishing that I was in Greece, experiencing 35 degrees, sitting with a pina colada on the beach!

A couple of my clients have just come back from their summer holiday for the year. Tanned, relaxed, in an excellent mood, and raring to get going again. Asking them and others their views on holidays and taking time out, the overwhelming response was "to relax and try not to think about work". This is from people of working age. Asking my 70-year-old parents the same question, it's about experiencing a new culture or environment, and changing the scenery from a quiet, retired life at home. We remember our holidays from a very young age, we spend the majority of the year saving up and looking forward to our next holiday, we meet new and different people when we are away, we eat different and exciting food, and we try different activities. We are usually very happy on holiday.

This also holds true regarding the UK weather. There is a marked difference in mood when the sun is shining and it's a pleasant day in comparison to a windy, rainy, grey day. Living in Henley, a tourist hotspot, I see this in action every weekend! When the sun is out, the pubs, restaurants, parks, and boat trips are full. On a grey day, local profits and mood levels are definitely down.

Is it the contrast with normal life and the chance to forget about your worries at home/work? Or are there physiological and psychological reactions in your body that happen when you are on holiday, when the weather is lovely, or if you are in a place you like?

Do you really need to go on holiday?

Research (and common sense) suggests we should certainly be thinking about booking our next trip away as soon as possible. An article in Forbes strongly suggests that taking a break from work is absolutely essential if you want to keep your employees, as it is integral to well-being, sustained productivity and high performance:

"A recent study by the World Health Organization (WHO) found that 745,000 people died in 2016 from heart disease and stroke due to long (working) hours. The research found that working 55 hours or more a week was associated with a 35% higher risk of stroke and a 17% higher risk of dying from heart disease than a workweek of 35 to 40 hours." (Forbes, 2021)

Another excellent article by Harvard Business Review suggests that taking holiday time unclutters your mind, allows you to catch up with lost sleep hours, reduces levels of stress hormones in your body, and reduces blood pressure:

"In a study of 749 women, researchers found that those who took vacation less than once every six years were eight times more likely to develop heart problems compared to those who went on vacation twice a year. Going on vacation can also lower your chances of dying from coronary heart disease, including lower blood sugar levels and improved HDL or 'good' cholesterol levels." (Zucker, 2023)

Physiological reactions in the body

So what is happening in our bodies when we relax on holiday in the sunshine?

Reduced stress hormones: Going on holiday in the sun has been linked to a reduction in stress hormones, such as cortisol. Sunlight exposure triggers the release of endorphins, often referred to as 'feel-good' hormones, which help counteract the negative effects of stress on the body. Endorphins promote relaxation, elevate mood, and contribute to an overall sense of well-being.

Vitamin D synthesis: Sun exposure is crucial for the production of vitamin D in our bodies. When our skin comes into contact with sunlight, it stimulates the synthesis of vitamin D from cholesterol. Vitamin D is essential for multiple physiological functions, including aiding in the absorption of calcium and phosphorus for healthy bones, regulating immune system function, and supporting cardiovascular health. Additionally, vitamin D has been found to play a role in the regulation of serotonin, a neurotransmitter that influences mood, appetite, and sleep.

Improved sleep quality: Sunlight exposure can also have a positive impact on our sleep quality. Exposure to natural light during the day helps to regulate our sleep-wake cycles, known as the circadian rhythm. This, in turn, improves the quality of our sleep, leading to better rest, increased alertness during the day, and improved overall cognitive function.

Increased serotonin levels: Sunlight exposure stimulates the release of serotonin in the brain. Serotonin is often referred to as the 'happy hormone' as it is associated with feelings of happiness, relaxation, and improved mood. Higher levels of serotonin are linked to reduced symptoms of depression and anxiety.

Enhanced immune system function: Moderate exposure to sunlight has been shown to positively influence the functioning of our immune system. Sunlight stimulates the production of certain immune cells, such as T cells and natural killer cells, which play a crucial role in defending the body against pathogens and fighting infections.

Psychological reactions

It's not just physical reactions that are important; spiritual reactions are as well.

Mental restoration: Holidays provide us with a chance to unwind, relax, and recharge. When we detach ourselves from the stresses of work and responsibilities, we allow our minds to rejuvenate. Engaging in enjoyable activities, exploring new places, and spending time with loved ones can enhance our mood, reduce anxiety, and increase overall happiness.

Cognitive flexibility: Stepping into a different environment during a holiday encourages cognitive flexibility. We become more open to new experiences, adapt to unfamiliar situations, and expand our perspectives. This mental flexibility gained during a holiday can have lasting impacts on our creativity, problem-solving abilities, and overall mental agility. Where do you think I came up with the idea for my business in the first place, many years ago now!!

Where is your happy place?

It doesn't necessarily need to be a holiday abroad that can help with physical and mental happiness and rejuvenation though. It could be in your favourite pub down the road when you meet up with friends, it could be that lovely place you like to take your dog for a walk, or it could even be your comfy, squishy chair in your lounge at home. Finding a place where you can instantly feel calm, safe, relaxed, and certainly happy, is an extremely important part of sustained happiness. Your haven. Your sanctuary.

"When people talk about their 'happy place,' it's usually a place that allows them to let go of daily pressures, reconnect with themselves at a soul level, and feel a sense of peace. It's here that you are able to express your values unencumbered – whether it's adventure, learning, or beauty – and do things that bring you joy." (Zucker, 2023)

Unravelling the meaning of haven

The concept of a haven varies for each individual. It could be a physical location – your cosy room, a comforting nook in your home, a secluded beach, or a picturesque garden. However, a haven is not merely confined to these external spaces. It can also manifest within ourselves – a mental sanctuary, where tranquillity is found in meditation, reflection, or engaging in a hobby that brings inner fulfilment.

The significance of feeling happy

As I have stated many times, happiness is the cornerstone of a fulfilling life. Recognising the importance of finding a place that brings us joy allows us to nurture our well-being. It is in these moments of happiness that we can truly unwind, rejuvenate, and recharge our energies. A haven should be a space where you can embrace the things that make you genuinely happy, whether it be singing, painting, reading, or spending quality time with loved ones.

The essence of safety

A haven should be a refuge, a place where you feel safe and protected. It should be a space that shields you from the worries, fears, and uncertainties of the outside world. Feeling secure within this haven allows you to let go of anxieties and fosters a sense of inner peace. It becomes a sanctuary where you can freely express yourself, where vulnerability is embraced, and where you can discover your authentic self.

Cultivating calmness

In our fast-paced, hectic lives, finding a haven that promotes calmness is crucial. This is a place where you can escape from the demands and pressures of daily life, a space that encourages mindfulness and facilitates self-reflection. Creating an environment that cultivates calmness – through soft lighting, comfortable furnishings, or natural elements – can significantly contribute to your overall well-being. It is within this calmness that clarity of thought emerges, paving the way for personal growth.

Time to relax and think

The modern world often leaves us little time for self-care, relaxation, and deep contemplation. Yet, finding a haven that allows you to unwind and think is vital for our mental and emotional well-being. It is in these moments of tranquillity that you can listen to your inner voice, connect with your aspirations, reflect on your journeys, and set new goals. A haven provides uninterrupted space, free from distractions, where you can explore your thoughts, dreams, and passions.

Summary

Firstly, going on holiday is more than just a temporary escape from daily life. It offers numerous psychological and physiological benefits. By providing a break from routine, reducing stress, promoting mental flexibility, and triggering positive chemical reactions in our bodies, holidays contribute to our overall health and well-being. These reactions include the reduction of stress hormones, the synthesis of vitamin D, increased serotonin levels, improved sleep quality, and enhanced immune system function. So, make sure to prioritise taking time off, exploring new destinations, and embracing the positive effects that a holiday can have on both your mind and your body.

Secondly, a haven serves as a sanctuary for our souls – a place where happiness, safety, calmness, relaxation, and thoughtful contemplation intertwine. Discovering such a place and nurturing it becomes a crucial part of our self-care and personal growth. So, take the time to find your haven, be it a physical location or a state of mind, and honour the importance of creating a space that brings you joy, peace, and the freedom to reflect upon life's meaningful moments. This is certainly not easy – especially if you have young children and a manic job, but even if you return to your chosen place for a few minutes in your head, this will help.

Action Time

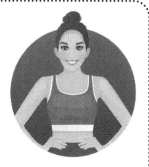

This is a written action.

1. Using the space on the following page, write a list of the places you would like to visit in the world – (please be realistic though!)

2. Prioritise them and assign a budget to each of them. This will form part of your 'big list' – more on this later!

3. Start to plan how you are going to work your way through them.

My examples: In the next seven years, I would like to visit Dubai, Croatia, Barbados, Japan, and Cornwall. Wow – I need to start saving!!

A bit of alone time

"Don't underestimate the value of Doing Nothing, of just going along, listening to all the things you can't hear, and not bothering."

Winnie the Pooh – A.A. Milne

One of the survey answers I received about happiness was "spending time on my own". This would not have been my first answer as I like to have people around me! But having some time to yourself is, in fact, more important for your mental well-being than it seems and perhaps I need to give it another try. In this chapter, we will explore how dedicating time to yourself can significantly contribute to personal happiness. If you are a parent of younger children, you may well read this chapter with another level of empathy for some alone time...

Understanding solitude

Although solitude can be considered negative when not self-chosen, according to an article on Medium.com by Thomas Oppong, the definition is: *"the intentional act of being alone, free from distractions and external influences."* It is a state of introspection, providing an opportunity to reconnect with oneself and recharge.

It allows you to step away from the noise and demands of everyday life, enabling introspection and self-reflection. This inner reflection helps individuals gain clarity, find inner peace, and adjust their perspective on life.

Benefits of time to yourself

Self-discovery and self-awareness: Spending time alone enables individuals to explore their thoughts, feelings, and aspirations. It provides an opportunity for self-discovery, allowing you to understand your values, desires, and needs better. This self-awareness is essential for finding true happiness. However, this isn't that easy to do!

I listened to a podcast by Stephen Warley titled 'How to Practice Self-Awareness'. It suggests some helpful tips to put this into practice. I found the most helpful activity was to take note of the most positive and the most negative feelings of the day to see if a pattern formed during the week.

As an example, today, I had the most positive feelings when I spent a fabulous hour with two of my clients that I have been training for years now and just laughing, dancing around the gym, and catching up on the gossip of the week whilst we were working out. My most negative feelings came when stuck in a traffic jam on the M25 with my children for 1.5 hours, whilst they were arguing and complaining. I felt anger and frustration, and contemplated pulling off to the side of the road and walking home! Being aware of your feelings and seeing if there are patterns that you can look to alter is a very good start!

Stress reduction and mental well-being: Me-time offers a much-needed break from the continuous stimulation and demands of daily life. Solitude provides an avenue for reducing stress, calming the mind, and restoring mental well-being. It allows space for reflection, healing, and rejuvenation. I have often spoken to friends and clients about the importance of taking time off for yourself, even if it is only an hour. However, the constant feedback about this is one of guilt. "I should be working, sorting the house, looking after the children etc..." We all have 101 things we should be getting on with, but I have often found that even taking five minutes out for myself makes me much more productive at work and home, and a more pleasant person to be around.

Boosting creativity and productivity: Solitude fosters a conducive environment for creativity and productivity. When the mind is free from external distractions, it can wander and explore new horizons. Time alone allows you to tap into your creative potential and find inspiration.

"There's a reason a lot of authors or artists want to go to a cabin in the woods or a private studio to work. Being alone with your thoughts gives your brain a chance to wander, which can help you become more creative." (Morin, 2017)

In Episode 4 of the podcast series *The One You Feed*, 'The Art of Stopping' by David Kundtz, he discusses the importance of exactly what you decide to give attention to in your life and how this makes a marked difference in your ability to enjoy it. He uses the analogy of 'the mountain of doing too much', explaining that humans can only do a certain amount each day or week, and everything we task ourselves to do can become overwhelming if we let it. We are programmed to continuously be busy and almost wear it as a badge of honour.

The practice of the 'art of stopping' means that for even a very short period of time, you sit down, close your eyes and **do nothing**. Doing nothing helps you to remember who you are and what you want: your goals. When you get up and get going again, there is more purpose. Stopping allows access to make decisions between what is important to us and what isn't – giving you the power to say no sometimes and having time to get off the treadmill of life and reflect.

This practice can be extremely hard to do with all the things going on in one's life, so David suggests starting by practising 'still points' – even if this is a few seconds at a time. Stop, close your eyes, be still, and have time to think and breathe. Pick a moment that will trigger your still point – when getting in your car at the end of your working day, when you finish an online meeting, when you have put the kids to bed. Destress and declutter your mind.

Implementing self-care practices

Prioritising time for yourself: Make a conscious effort to create a schedule that includes dedicated time for self-care. Whether it's a few minutes each day or longer periods during the week, setting aside this time allows you to focus on activities that bring you joy and fulfilment. I always find a relaxing soak in a bubble bath is a very helpful and lovely way to spend 30 minutes.

Engaging in activities you love: Identify activities that make you happy and dedicate time to them. It could be reading, writing, painting, taking walks in nature, practising mindfulness, or indulging in a hobby. Engaging in activities that align with your passions recharges your energy and cultivates happiness. My favourite activity when I know I need a bit of self-care is to bake – yes, knowing me, it will be low sugar, probably have some kind of fruit or vegetable in it, and some protein powder for an extra boost, but I love the feeling of creating something from scratch with a few things from the cupboard. My children are slightly less convinced!

Unplug and disconnect: In an increasingly connected world, it is vital to disconnect from technology and social media occasionally. Unplugging, even for short durations, helps reduce mental clutter, allowing for a more profound connection with oneself and the present moment.

Summary

In the pursuit of happiness, dedicating time to oneself should not be underestimated. Solitude and self-care provide an opportunity for self-discovery, reflection, and rejuvenation. By embracing moments of solitude and engaging in self-care activities, you can nourish your mind, body, and spirit, ultimately finding greater happiness and well-being in your life.

Action Time

This is a written action.

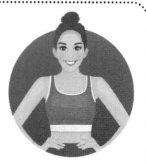

1. Using the space below, write down three tasks in your day that are daily habits.

2. Try and think if you could add the practice of enjoying a 'still moment' around these tasks.

My example: Dropping the kids off to school – before I restart the car, I just close my eyes, sit still for 30 seconds, and enjoy the inner peace before I crack on with my day.

Sleepy bunnies

"Twinkle, twinkle, little star,
How I wonder what you are!
Up above the world so high,
Like a diamond in the sky.
Twinkle, twinkle, little star,
How I wonder where you are!"

19th-century English lullaby

I cannot tell you how many times I ask my clients, my children, my husband and my friends how well they slept. It makes such an enormous difference to their productivity and their mood, and therefore how they are going to react to me on any given day. In our fast-paced modern world, it can be all too easy to sacrifice sleep in favour of work, socialising, or simply trying to fit more hours into the day. However, neglecting sleep can have an extremely detrimental effect on our physical and mental well-being. In this chapter, we will explore the importance of sleep, what happens to our bodies during this crucial period of rest, and techniques to enjoy a good night's sleep.

The importance of sleep

I could harp on about this for many chapters, as I believe so strongly about the power of sleep, but I have noted the fundamentals which follow. Sleep is a biological process that plays a vital role in maintaining our overall health. Not only does it allow our bodies to rest and recharge, but it also supports proper cognitive function, emotional well-being, and physical performance. Adequate sleep promotes a strong immune system, enhances memory and learning, regulates mood and emotions, improves creativity, and boosts problem-solving abilities. There are many published books that talk entirely about the importance of sleep. Here are two of my favourites:

The Sleep Revolution by Arianna Huffington explains how sleep is so critical and that it isn't just about feeling better in the morning, it's a way of improving your work performance, health, and even your personal relationships.

Similarly, *Sleep Smarter* by Shawn Stevenson uses a very practical approach to improving the quality of your sleep, and why maintaining a healthy body and mind is crucial for getting a good night's sleep.

"Sleep is as important for good health as diet and exercise. Good sleep improves your brain performance, mood, and health." (News in Health, 2021)

I have come across a number of people who confidently claim they function perfectly well with less than seven to eight hours of sleep per night. However, on close analysis, it seems that aspects of their health and well-being have suffered due to a continuous habit of averaging less than their body and mind need. It has formed into a habit that their body and mind are currently putting up with, rather than thriving on. For this to be tested, you do need to be honest with yourself! You operate on five hours per night, but are you are quite snappy and cranky later in the afternoon? Do you rely on caffeine? Do you feel less alert in the afternoon? Does your skin tend to look a little sallow? Are you suffering from high blood pressure and weight gain? If you answered yes to a chunk of these, are you truly OK with less than seven hours' sleep in reality? I think the answer would be no!

I recently conducted a small sleep study with some of my clients to see if their sleep could be improved and what was causing the sleep problems in the first place. I worked with them for a four-week period and asked them to note their sleep each morning after waking. If they used a devise such as an Apple watch to track their sleep patterns, I also looked at this data. From interviewing them and looking at noted results, I identified two main themes: Waking up multiple times in the night, and taking ages to get to sleep. The reasons varied quite substantially, but are listed as follows:

- Children waking them up

- House noises and partner snoring

- Room temperature – too hot or too cold

- Alcohol consumption before going to bed

- Hormones – monthly menstrual cycle or menopause

- Needing a pee in the night

- Eating too late in the evening

Below are three examples of clients from that study with whom I worked with to understand a pattern, then tried to resolve.

Case study 1: David – alcohol

David works very hard and has a high-powered and stressful job. He tries a number of different ways to relax at the end of his day, including having a lovely, warm bath and good levels of exercise, but he is partial to a few glasses of wine at the end of the day as well. After looking at patterns of sleep, in conjunction with his daily food/drink consumption, there is a distinct pattern between the evenings he didn't sleep well and the amount of alcohol consumed that evening. After a week's trial of not drinking as much or any alcohol, there was a marked improvement in quality of sleep and length of time staying asleep. Although falling asleep can be a little easier after consuming alcohol, it is being processed in your body and will disrupt your system's normal patterns, causing a disturbed night's sleep.

"On the face of it, drinking an alcoholic beverage before bed may seem like a great way to get to sleep. After all, ethanol's depressant effects on the CNS lead to drowsiness and reduce the time it takes to fall asleep, irrespective of how much ethanol has been consumed. However, once

asleep, ethanol can disrupt normal sleep patterns so that the quality of sleep, measured by the time spent in REM and non-REM sleep and total time asleep is reduced. Non-REM deep sleep is considered as regenerative, mainly due to the release of growth hormone, and, although this type of sleep is increased when ethanol is consumed, growth hormone secretion by the pituitary gland is decreased". (Roehrs & Roth, 2001)

Case study 2: Jane – noise

Jane lives in a busy household with her husband, children and their dog, in a lovely, but creaky house. It is rarely quiet and the family's sleep patterns are all different. Since becoming a mother, Jane has found she has become a very light sleeper and the slightest bit of noise wakes her up. She is on edge to react if need be, then finds it hard to get back to sleep. Her husband snores, her (older) children often go to bed later than her, and her dog sleeps in their room and can move around in the night. The solution? To try ear plugs. The only thing preventing Jane from a restful night was the noise so we had to reduce it. The correct ear plugs needed to be found to fit comfortably and not fall out in the night, but this has so far worked very well.

Case study 3: Sarah – hormones

Since a young age, Sarah has experienced an uncomfortable and painful monthly menstrual cycle. She is still young and hasn't had children yet but finds that she struggles to sleep for an entire week a month. We looked at a number of factors to see what could be changed to help in this week. Exercise definitely helps and when Sarah is physically tired as well as mentally, she definitely sleeps better. However, we found that when her body temperature was regulated more effectively, this helped. Try and ensure your room is a slightly lower temperature than the rest of the house, layer your bed clothes so you can remove or add layers as you need to, and ensure your PJs are made from a breathable, cotton material. These slight amends kept Sarah more comfortable overnight and so aided a more restful sleep.

"Your body temperature dips a bit just before your ovary releases an egg. Then, 24 hours after the egg's release, your temperature rises and stays up for several days. Before ovulation, a woman's BBT averages between 97°F (36.1°C) and 97.5°F (36.4°C). After ovulation, it rises to 97.6°F (36.4°C) to 98.6°F (37°C)." (www.peacehealth.org)

What happens when we sleep

Sleep is a complex process consisting of various stages that our bodies cycle through repeatedly, typically in a 90-minute sequence for adults. These stages can be broadly classified into two categories: rapid eye movement (REM) sleep and non-REM sleep.

Non-REM sleep comprises three stages: N1 (light sleep) where we transition between wakefulness and sleep, N2 (intermediate sleep) characterised by deeper relaxation, and N3 (deep sleep) when our bodies undergo significant restoration and rejuvenation. REM sleep, which occurs later in the sleep cycle, is associated with vivid dreaming and crucial mental and emotional processing.

During sleep, our bodies engage in important physiological processes. These include tissue repair, hormone regulation, consolidation of memory, and strengthening of the immune system. Additionally, sleep provides an opportunity for the brain to clear out metabolic waste, promoting overall cognitive health.

"During deep sleep, your body works to repair muscle, organs, and other cells. Chemicals that strengthen your immune system start to circulate in your blood. You spend about a fifth of your night's sleep in deep sleep." (Web MD, 2021)

Consequences of sleep deprivation

Insufficient sleep or poor sleep quality can have serious consequences for our overall well-being. In the short term, it can lead to feelings of fatigue, lack of focus, forgetfulness, decreased alertness, and impaired judgement. Prolonged sleep deprivation can increase the risk of chronic conditions such as obesity, diabetes, heart disease, and mental health disorders like anxiety and depression. It can also compromise our immune system, increase the likelihood of accidents, and negatively impact relationships, work performance, and overall quality of life.

Sleep techniques

But what if we are struggling to get to sleep or stay asleep? Below are some techniques for helping to get a better night's sleep – many of these were tried and tested with my clients in my sleep study, and some I have used time and time again with my family and myself. However, these will not work for people with a sleep-related clinical diagnosis.

A set bedtime routine: Establish a relaxing pre-sleep routine to signal to your body that it's time to unwind. Engage in activities such as reading a book, taking a warm bath, or practising relaxation techniques like deep breathing or meditation. This is usually what we like to establish with our children, but it's no different for adults.

Your room temperature: This ideally should be between about 19 degrees and 21 degrees. People often have bedrooms a lot hotter than this, but this can make you wake up in the night.

Sleep spray: This is a great little trick for training your system to think 'bedtime'. You smell a spray which usually contains the calming scent of lavender and this triggers the habit of relaxing and preparing to sleep. I have found the best one is from the brand This Works.

Pillow and mattress comfort: Double-check that it's not your old and saggy mattress or pillow that is causing the problem. Mattresses should be changed, on average, every eight to ten years. When was the last time you changed yours?

Screen time before bed: Mobile phones and iPads have a 'night-time' mode for a reason. The light of the screen disturbs your melatonin production and can falsely keep you awake. Switch your phone to night-time mode from about 10 pm and try hard not to look at your screen for at least 30 minutes before you close your eyes to go to sleep.

Eating too near to bedtime: Research suggests that you should try to finish eating approximately 1.5 – 2 hours before going to bed. Your digestive system takes a lot of energy and effort to digest your meal and if vital energy is taken up with digestion as opposed to calming your brain at the end of the day, you will definitely not sleep as soundly.

Consistency of setting your bedtime: bodies and brains like routine (our circadian rhythm). If you try to set your bedtime for around the same time each evening, a correct habit will be formed and your sleep will be improved. For example, try to start your bedtime routine from 10:30 pm, be asleep by 11 pm and set your alarm for 6:30 am, every day; your system will thank you for it.

Hydration (needing a pee in the night): If you are constantly waking in the night for a pee, this can disturb your sleep pattern completely. Some medications can exacerbate this, but if there is no underlying reason that should be discussed with your doctor, you may just be drinking too much right at the end of the day.

Relaxation techniques: If you are struggling to get to sleep, my favourite technique is to listen to an audio book (one that you know well) or a sleep-specific hypnotherapy session. I find this a guaranteed way to drift off to sleep very quickly.

Children disturbing your sleep: The only one I am struggling to find an answer for!!! If you have tiny little ones and they are waking up in the night and waking you up, from one parent to another I can tell you this; it is a little overwhelming at the time, but it will get better and you will get your sleep back! Try and go to bed early each evening, and keep their and your bedtime consistent.

Summary

Sleep is a vital component of maintaining our overall health and well-being. Understanding the importance of sleep, its various stages, and the consequences of deprivation can help us prioritise it in our lives. By implementing techniques for a good night's sleep, such as establishing a routine, creating a relaxing sleep environment, and adopting healthy pre-sleep habits, we can optimise our sleep quality and reap the many benefits that come with it. Please be assured, a good night's sleep is the foundation for a happier, healthier life.

Action Time

This is a practical action.

If you find you are struggling to get to sleep, I would like you to try even one of the suggestions in the above chapter.

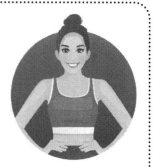

1. On an iPhone: Go to the 'Health' app on your phone and find the 'sleep' section.

2. Set your sleep to allow for at least seven hours.

3. You can also set an alarm to wake you at the moment your phone comes out of sleep mode.

My example: My sleep setting is from 10 pm to 6 am. I have a 15-minute wind-down period in which my phone will prompt me at 9:45 pm to start the bedtime routine. I go upstairs and get myself prepared for bed, so I am ideally in bed for when my phone goes into sleep mode – my applications will not disturb me but the phone is still switched on so I will receive a call in the night in an emergency. At 6 am, my phone wishes me 'Good Morning' and returns to normal lighting and functions. This has helped me stay in my routine and get enough sleep. I have a very busy and active day between 6 am – 10 pm so definitely need this.

1C – HAPPINESS AND WORK

It's all work, work, work...

"Hi ho, hi ho, it's off to work we go..."

Walt Disney's *Snow White and the Seven Dwarfs*

The next couple of chapters focus more on happiness within the workplace, but many of the principles I discuss here can be carried through to your personal life as well. We spend over a third of our life at work – on average nearly 90,000 hours across our working lifetime (Gettysburg.edu) – so we should at least try to find some joy in as many of these hours as possible!

I consider myself extremely lucky and in the minority when it comes to how I feel about my job and I remind myself of this frequently. Although the working hours are very long per day, I love what I do and I genuinely don't suffer from feelings of negativity or ever dread 'going in'. What I do isn't easy though and running your own company is relentless, but the satisfaction levels gained from my job are very high. However, this might not be the case for you and it's certainly not the case for most other people either. But what to do about it?

"A whopping 80% of us here in the UK are NOT happy with our current career or job role and, surprisingly, those of us with some of the highest earning potential are in fact some of the least happy people." (Open Study College, 2023)

Finding purpose and meaning in your work

I read an interesting article from the careers guidance company 80,000 Hours – with that name, they assume fewer hours than others suggest (I like that!). After gathering evidence from over 60 research pieces, the company found six major factors contributing to having your dream job, which are what you should aim for when deciding on a job or judging your current job. It was not purely about getting paid as much as you possibly can for the hours you work:

1. Work that is engaging (freedom, clear tasks, variety, feedback)

2. Work that helps others

3. Work you are good at

4. Work with supportive colleagues

5. Work that doesn't have major negatives (e.g. a long commute, very long hours, unfair pay)

6. Work that fits with the rest of your life

Taking the above into consideration, the good news is that it's not too late to find purpose and meaning in your work! Here are some steps you can take to inject passion and meaning back into your career.

Think about your passions and interests

What drives you? What do you enjoy doing in your spare time? By understanding your passions and interests, you can begin to understand what you find meaningful. If you're struggling to find an answer, consider trying new hobbies or activities to see what resonates with you.

I am lucky enough to work with a gentleman called Julian, who used to work in the marketing industry in a senior position at a high flying agency – a mad, interesting world but with crazy hours, very high stress levels, and huge expectations on staff. Julian took the call a number of years ago to follow his dreams, re-qualify and start his own business as a sports massage therapist, personal trainer, class instructor and acupuncturist. He has a completely different lifestyle now, with a very worthwhile and satisfying job. He helps many people from different walks of life and works this around what he wants to do rather than what he is expected to do. (fitterlonger.com)

Identify your strengths

What are your natural abilities? What do you excel at? When you're working in a role that plays to your strengths, you're more likely to feel fulfilled. Consider taking a personality test or a strengths finder quiz to help you identify your skills. Have a read of the next chapter, 'Understanding Your Personality Profile', for further info on personality tests – they are interesting, very helpful, and will provide some clear insight into your natural or learnt strengths. When you are in a role that fights against this, it can be very stressful and not long-term sustainable.

The bestselling book *How to Enjoy Your Life and Your Job*, by the amazing Dale Carnegie, provides guidance on how to get more out of your working day by creating more energy for it, as well as how to improve your personal relationships. For example, changing your attitude towards criticism and how to deliver criticism to others, will ensure your day is much happier. Not only will you get much better results from others, but you will learn more yourself from responding more positively.

Consider a career change

A little scary to think about at first, but if you've tried to find purpose in your current role and it's just not working, it might be time for a change. Consider exploring other industries or roles that align with your passions and interests. A shift in career can be a scary prospect, but it can also be incredibly rewarding.

I would like to introduce you to James Thomas. The lovely James co-owns and runs (with his wife) a very successful dog walking and sitting service called Dogs of Henley, and has been for nearly 10 years now. He is fit as a fiddle, walks for hours every day, gets up at 5:30 am every morning, and his house is filled with little hounds all day! He literally loves what he does, would never change it for the world and, like me, considers himself extremely lucky. James, however, used to sit at a desk all day on the phone for a recruitment consultancy. He was successful at his job, but hated it. He is an outdoor kind of man and even though it was a daunting move, he did it and hasn't looked back!

Invest in your personal growth

Personal growth and development can be hugely fulfilling. Seek out training opportunities or mentorship programs to learn new skills and grow professionally. By building up your knowledge and expertise, you'll be better equipped to make a meaningful contribution in your role.

Since changing career over six years ago from the advertising and recruitment industry, I gained personal training and class instructor qualifications, then over time have added Pilates, mental health first aid, counselling and nutrition coach qualifications. They have vastly added to my skill set, allowed me to offer additional services to my clients and gym members, giving me and my work an additional level of professionalism and expertise. These qualifications have also helped with my personal growth, as I now understand more about how human bodies and minds work, including my own!

Fitting work around life, not life around work

I spent many years of my working life in an industry where it was definitely 'life around work' – crazy hours, crazy stress levels, poor pay, dictated to by senior staff/clients, and high expectations to socialise after work with colleagues/clients. It was a massive learning curve as a graduate and an amazing start to working life due to the amount I was exposed to, but my goodness, it takes it out of everyone who works in the advertising and marketing world, and still does! Of course, we weren't saving lives, but with certain jobs you have to make a decision to sacrifice some or nearly all of your social and home life to be able to do it – doctors and nurses on call being the most obvious example.

However, this is not usually the case for the vast majority of jobs. Hours are set, tasks and expectations for the day/week/year are clear, and the pay cheque is constant. So why do we never have time to fit in what we want to do, rather than simply what we are paid to do? I would suggest it's all about correct scheduling.

But I don't have time! Life scheduling

I cannot tell you how many times I hear, "Yeah, I know I should, but I don't have the time…" However, there is definitely some truth in the saying, "If you really want to do something, you will make time." So, if we are all busy and struggling for time to fit in some exercise, for example, then how do some people manage it? It's all about correct scheduling!

First, let's talk about the importance of scheduling. When you create a schedule, you're essentially setting priorities and assigning time to activities that matter most. This helps you to be more intentional with your time and can prevent you from feeling overwhelmed or scattered. There is no way at all I would be able to do or remember even half of what I need to do in a week, let alone a day, without the following tips;

Tips for creating an effective schedule

Write everything down: Start by making a list of all the tasks, events, appointments, and other commitments that you have throughout the day or week. This can help you to see where you might have conflicts or overlapping priorities.

Use a calendar or planner: Once you have everything written down, transfer it to a calendar or planner. This can be a digital tool (like Google Calendar) or a physical book. The point is to have everything in one place so you can see the big picture.

Prioritise: Decide what items on your list are most important, and assign a specific time to them in your schedule. Be realistic about what you can accomplish in the allotted time, and don't forget to include breaks and downtime for activities like exercise, relaxation, and socialising.

Stick to it: Once you've created your schedule, commit to following it as closely as possible. Of course, there will be times when things come up and you need to be flexible, but try to stay on track as much as possible.

Benefits of scheduling your life

Reduce stress and anxiety: Having a clear plan for how you're going to spend your time can help alleviate feelings of stress and anxiety. When you know what's coming up and have a plan for how you're going to handle it, you're less likely to feel overwhelmed.

Improve time management skills: By scheduling your time effectively, you're able to practice time management, which will help you get more done in less time. This can free up time for other activities that you enjoy, like spending time with family and friends.

Promote self-care: When you're intentional about scheduling time for activities such as exercise, meditation, and relaxation, you're prioritising your own health and well-being. This can help you to be more productive and focused in the long run.

Enhance productivity: When you have a plan in place for how you're going to use your time, you're less likely to waste it on unimportant or non-essential tasks. This can help to increase your productivity and focus.

Getting away from your desk

Even if you are in a job role you enjoy, all of us need breaks in our day, especially if you have a computer-based role. The last section looks at the importance of stepping away from your desk at points during the day and offers practical advice on how to do this efficiently and effectively.

Physical and mental health benefits

Prolonged periods of desk work can lead to various physical and mental health issues. Sitting for long hours can contribute to poor posture, muscle imbalances, and an increased risk of cardiovascular problems. Taking regular breaks, including brief walks or simple stretching exercises, can promote blood circulation, reduce muscle tension, and alleviate physical discomfort. Furthermore, stepping away from your desk allows your mind to rest and recharge, combating mental fatigue, and enhancing focus and concentration when you return.

Creativity and problem-solving

Being constantly tethered to our desks can hinder our ability to think creatively and solve problems. Immersing ourselves in a different environment, whether it be taking a walk, visiting a coffee shop, or even finding a cosy spot in the office lounge, can stimulate new perspectives and fresh ideas. By giving our minds the freedom to wander and take in new stimuli, we tap into our creative reserves and improve our problem-solving abilities.

When I was in advertising, I worked for a lovely agency in Brisbane, Australia for a while. We were given a new brief by one of our most important clients at the time, Tabcorp Casino Group, and it was the biggest campaign they had done for several years so wanted to make a huge statement. The campaign was for an international poker tournament they were running across two of their biggest casinos in the country. Instead of briefing my creative team in the office, as per usual, I set up a poker game with professionals so they could immerse us in the world of poker! They taught us what it feels like to play, to win or lose, and to how speak to the people at the centre of the world of poker. It was the most successful campaign Tabcorp Casino Group ever ran, and secured our relationship with them for many years to come.

Relationship building and collaboration

Getting away from your desk allows for valuable opportunities to foster relationships and engage in beneficial collaborations. Taking breaks with co-workers or networking with others outside your department can lead to new connections and enhance teamwork. Informal conversations during a break often spark creative discussions and fresh insights. Building relationships and collaborating with colleagues in a relaxed setting can contribute to a more vibrant and supportive work environment.

Summary

Finding purpose and meaning in your work is a journey, not a destination. It takes time and effort to explore your passions and interests, and to find the role that fits you best. But with the right mindset and a willingness to put in the work, you can find a career that feels both fulfilling, meaningful, and brings you happiness.

Plus, while it may seem counter-intuitive, taking breaks and getting away from our desks is crucial for maintaining a healthy work environment, achieving optimal productivity, and improving overall well-being. By scheduling correctly and prioritising our physical and mental health, embracing creativity, and fostering relationships, as well as finding a work-life balance, we can enhance our professional performance and lead happier, more fulfilled lives. So, remember to step away from your desk, recharge, and return with renewed energy and focus – your mind, body, and colleagues will thank you.

Action Time

This is a practical action.

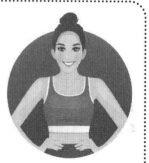

1. Set reminders on your computer calendar or on your phone to get up and move every two hours. This can be for a few seconds or a few minutes, but at the very least, stand up, take a deep breath, and look away from your computer.

2. Try this for a month and see if this helps you.

My example: Writing this book has meant that I have been on my computer much more than I usually am – so I have taken my own advice and set reminders on my phone!

Understanding your personality profile

I have chosen to add this topic because if you understand yourself and others more, it will make your life much easier, and therefore you will be much happier. In my recruitment days, we used personality profiling techniques all the time – they proved very useful to understand how a job candidate would likely fit with a new team and company. I have been profiled many times and I have always found it extremely helpful to understand how I will react to situations and how to manage others in a more effective way. This chapter explains what personality profiling is and how you can use this knowledge to be a happier person at work and at home.

Understanding ourselves and others is key to building harmonious relationships and maximising our potential. One popular tool for personality profiling is the DISC model. This categorises individuals into four primary behavioural styles: Dominance (D), Influence (I), Steadiness (S), and Conscientiousness/Conformity (C). In this chapter, we explore the benefits of DISC profiling and how understanding personality profiles can promote happiness both in our personal lives and professional environments.

Self-awareness and personal growth

DISC profiling provides valuable insights into our own behavioural preferences. By understanding our own tendencies, strengths, and areas for improvement, we can develop greater self-awareness and work towards personal growth. For example, if we have a dominant (D) behavioural style, we may recognise our assertiveness and take steps to balance it with active listening and incorporating others' perspectives. This self-awareness fosters personal development and helps us become happier individuals.

	HIGH DOMINANT STYLE	HIGH INFLUENCING STYLE	HIGH STEADY STYLE	HIGH CONSCIENTIOUS STYLE
Tends to Act	Assertive	Persuasive	Patient	Contemplative
When in Conflict, this Style	Demands Action	Attacks	Complies	Avoids
Needs	Control	Approval	Routine	Standards
Primary Drive	Independence	Interaction	Stability	Correctness
Preferred Tasks	Challenging	People related	Scheduled	Structured
Comfortable with	Being decisive	Social friendliness	Being part of a team	Order and planning
Personal Strength	Problem solver	Encourager	Supporter	Organiser
Strength Overextended	Preoccupation on goals over people	Speaking without thinking	Procrastination in addressing change	Over analyzing everything
Personal Limitation	Too direct and intense	Too disorganised and nontraditional	Too indecisive and indirect	Too detailed and impersonal
Personal Wants	Control, Variety	Approval, Less Structure	Routine, Harmony	Standards, Logic
Personal Fear	Losing	Rejection	Sudden Change	Being Wrong
Blind Spots	Being held accountable	Follow through on commitments	Embracing need for change	Struggle to make decisions without overanalyzing
Needs to Work on	Empathy, Patience	Controlling emotions, Follow through	Being assertive when pressured	Worrying less about everything
Measuring Maturity	Giving up control	Objectively handling rejection	Standing up for self when confronted	Not being defensive when criticised
Under Stress May Become	Dictatorial, Critical	Sarcastic, Superficial	Submissive, Indecisive	Withdrawn, Headstrong
Measures Worth by	Impact or results, Track record	Acknowledgments, Compliments	Compatibility, Contributions	Precision, Accuracy, Quality of results

https://actioncoach.co.uk/free-disc-profile

Enhanced communication and interpersonal skills

Understanding the DISC personality profiles of others paves the way for improved communication and stronger relationships. By recognising each behavioural style's communication preferences, we can adjust our approach to effectively connect with different individuals. For instance, an influencer (I) may respond well to enthusiasm and collaboration, while a conscientious (C) person may appreciate thorough analysis and attention to detail. This adaptability in communication promotes understanding, reduces conflicts, and contributes to happier interactions both at home and at work.

Building productive teams

DISC profiling is invaluable for creating productive and cohesive teams in the workplace. When forming teams, considering the diverse mix of personality styles can lead to enhanced collaboration and synergy. By leveraging the strengths of different profiles, teams can excel in problem-solving, decision-making, and achieving common goals. For example, a team consisting of dominants (D) for leadership, influencers (I) for relationship-building, steadiness (S) for maintaining team morale, and conscientiousness (C) for attention to detail can create a well-rounded and harmonious dynamic. A happy and productive team environment promotes job satisfaction and overall well-being.

Conflict resolution and emotional intelligence

DISC profiling equips individuals with tools for effective conflict resolution and emotional intelligence. By understanding the behavioural patterns and preferences of others, we can better navigate conflicts and find mutually agreeable solutions. Recognising the motivations and fears associated with each behavioural style allows us to approach conflicts with empathy and understanding. This leads to constructive conversations, reduced tension, and ultimately, increased happiness for all parties involved.

A case study

This can be quite complex to understand if you don't have a case study to look at. I have been DISC profiled recently, so thought I would share the fundamentals with you to bring it to life a little more. For those who know me, have a read and see if you agree!!

The following chart is a summary of the words that describe my personality profile. 'I' is my prominent trait – I am a complete people-person and being with others in a social environment is most important to me. There is also a summary of my strengths, work style tendencies, most effective environments, and potential areas for improvement. It's quite uncanny how accurate it is – I have to take the rough with the smooth and definitely need to work on my patience levels!

DISC Focus	D Problems / Tasks	I People	S Pace or Environment	C Procedures
Needs	Challenges to solve, Authority	Social relationships, Friendly environment	Systems, Teams, Stable environment	Rules to follow, Data to analyze
Emotions	Anger, Impatience	Optimism, Trust	Patience, Non-Expressions	Fear, Concern
Fears	Being taken advantage of/lack of control	Being left out, loss of social approval	Sudden change/loss of stability and security	Being criticized/loss of accuracy and quality

I am an 'I,D' profile. The wording used to describe are:

I – Enthusiastic, persuasive, optimistic, emotional, impulsive, gregarious

D – Assertive, competitive, determined, self-reliant

S – Alert, eager, flexible, mobile

C – Autonomous, independent, firm, stubborn

Rebecca's Strengths

- You are a very active agent in all that you do.

- You demand a high performance from yourself and others.

- You have excellent presentation skills when dealing with groups. You bring a poised, confident, and engaging message to any audience.

- You are excellent at initiating activity and providing direction for the team or organisation.

- You are able to make decisions quickly and to take the credit or blame for the outcome of decisions.

- You have a strong tendency to work toward making things happen, rather than waiting for things to happen.

- You tend to set high goals, then work hard with people to achieve those goals.

Rebecca's Work Style Tendencies

- You are a self-starter with a strong competitive edge.

- You are able to delegate, while maintaining control over activities within the project.

- You tend to be a 'multi-tasker', capable of juggling several projects simultaneously.

- Your pace of personal operation is faster than that of many people.

- You are able to think quickly on your feet – you can react, adjust, or modify your behaviour in a variety of situations.

- You set high operational goals for yourself and others, and expect all involved to provide maximum effort.

- You have the ability to inspire others to reach their maximum potential.

Rebecca Tends to Be Most Effective in Environments That Provide

- A responsive team with which to work and associate.

- Direct answers to questions.

- Responsibilities requiring a high degree of decisiveness.

- A variety of challenging assignments with high-stakes opportunities for success.

- A workplace that frees you from many details and heavy supervision.

- An arena for you to verbalise your ideas and opinions.

- Assignments involving the motivation and persuasion of a network of people.

Rebecca's Potential Areas for Improvement

- You may become somewhat angry or belligerent when under pressure, or when threatened.

- You could be a bit more willing to share talents in order to help others develop professionally. You may tend to be a bit too self-serving.

- You may sometimes take an 'ends justify the means' approach.

- You may become impatient, especially when dealing with slower-moving or slower-thinking people.

- You may need to lower project expectations a bit in light of real-world constraints.

- You may be a selective listener, at times hearing only what you want to hear.

- You may not always verbalise the complete story and tend to consciously withhold some information.

Summary

DISC profiling provides a valuable framework for understanding ourselves and others, enhancing communication, building productive teams, and promoting harmonious relationships. By recognising and appreciating the strengths and preferences of different behavioural styles, we enable personal growth, foster effective communication, and create a positive and collaborative environment both in our personal lives and professional settings. Embracing the insights provided by DISC profiling allows us to navigate challenges with greater ease, leading to increased happiness and fulfilment. So, take the time to explore your personality profile and embrace the power of understanding for a happier and more harmonious life.

Action Time

This is a practical action.

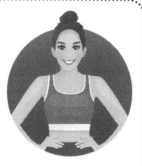

1. Look up one of the DISC profiling companies that offer a free trial or basic tool.

2. Fill in the details as requested and see what your DISC profile suggests.

3. Take note of what is being said and notice if there is anything about your profile that will help you manage or interact with others to make your and their lives happier.

My examples: There are many companies that offer DISC profiling services. Companies I have used before are Thomas International and Insights; even Tony Robbins has a DISC profiling tool on his website! The above profiling report was from DISCstyles™ Online Report, Action Coach UK.

Have a chat to my coach, Mark Van Rol. He is fabulous and will certainly help you with this: markvanrol.actioncoach.co.uk

Let's be SMART about this

*"What man actually needs is not a tensionless state,
but rather the striving and struggling for some goal worthy of him."*

Viktor E. Frankl
Austrian neurologist, psychiatrist and Holocaust survivor

In our journey towards personal and professional growth, setting goals is a fundamental step. However, not all goals are created equal, and this is where SMART goals come into play. SMART is an acronym for Specific, Measurable, Achievable, Relevant, and Time-bound. With my personal trainer hat on, this is a fundamental part of what I work on with my clients and it is essential to success and progress. I cannot stress the importance of setting goals in your life, but making them SMART will give you a much higher success rate. In this chapter, we will explore what SMART goals are, how they are used, and why they are essential in creating a clear path to success.

Specific: Setting a clear target

The first characteristic of a SMART goal is specificity. This means defining your goal in a clear and detailed manner. Rather than setting a vague goal like "improve my fitness", a SMART goal would be "participate in a half marathon within six months, running at least five times a week and gradually increasing mileage". By being specific, you provide yourself with a clear target to work towards, which makes it easier to plan and take action.

Measurable: Tracking progress and success

A SMART goal must be measurable, meaning it should include quantifiable criteria that allow you to track your progress. For example, if your goal is to save money, a specific and measurable goal could be "save £200 per month for six months". This allows you to track your progress and determine whether you are on track to achieve your goal. Measurable goals provide a sense of achievement and motivation as you witness your progress over time.

Achievable: Realistic and attainable

One key aspect of a SMART goal is that it must be achievable. Setting goals that are overly ambitious or unrealistic can lead to frustration and lack of motivation. A SMART goal is a balance between ambition and feasibility. It should stretch you out of your comfort zone but still be within the realm of possibility. By setting achievable goals, you increase your chances of success and maintain consistency in working towards them.

Relevant: Aligning goals with your values

A SMART goal should be relevant to your overall aspirations, values, and priorities. It should align with your long-term vision and be meaningful to you. Setting relevant goals ensures that you stay focused on what truly matters to you and avoids wasting time and energy on pursuits that don't contribute to your larger objectives. The relevance of a goal motivates and inspires you to take consistent action towards its achievement.

Time-bound: Setting deadlines and creating accountability

The final characteristic of a SMART goal is being time-bound, meaning it has a specific deadline. Without a set time frame, goals can easily fall by the wayside or be indefinitely postponed. By setting deadlines for our goals, we create a sense of urgency and accountability. For example, setting a deadline to complete a project within a month helps us break it down into manageable tasks and stay focused on a timeline. Time-bound goals provide a framework for planning and prioritising our actions, increasing our productivity and efficiency.

"First, a S.M.A.R.T. goal helps to give you an objective. In doing this, you are able to identify strengths and weaknesses. Second, a S.M.A.R.T. goal provides motivation to succeed. When you know where the goal line is, you'll want to work to meet or beat it. Third, a good S.M.A.R.T. goal, while attainable, will also be challenging and force you out of your comfort zone. Ultimately, the S.M.A.R.T. goal is a useful tool to remain focused in attaining a goal." (Leonard & Watts, 2022)

Let me show you a couple of examples of setting SMART goals. These are two of my personal training clients, and are physical exercise and nutrition related, but SMART goals can be related to any goal you are looking to achieve in your life.

Example 1 – Mark

(Mid 50s, 5ft 8", BMI normal) Mark would like to be able to run 10km. Three months ago, we ran a 5km race together and this was his first ever competitive race. He managed it in a respectable time of 34 minutes. He had no adverse effects from the race and, in fact, enjoyed the morning a lot more than he thought he was going to! He even received a fabulous medal at the end of it, for his efforts! He is now keen to double this and be able to finish a 10km race at the same location as it is flat and familiar. Let's see if we can make this SMART for Mark:

- Specific – Mark has stated the exact length of race he wants to achieve and the location. We look up the next 10km race at that location. It's in six months' time. He also wants to finish in one hour.

- Measurable – The length of the race is 10km and it will be measured by if he finishes, the time he takes, and if he remains injury-free during and after.

- Achievable – Mark is already fit enough to run 5km and we have six months to work on this together. Although not a breeze, this will be perfectly achievable, if he remains injury-free, in good health, and is able to attend his training sessions.

- Relevant – Mark is very keen to progress his running abilities and was highly motivated with the 5km race. This is a relevant and worthwhile goal for him.

- Time-bound – We have six months to complete this goal. There is an external deadline that we are working towards. It's very important this is set, or the goal could just drift and never be completed.

Example 2 – Mary

(Early 30s, 5ft 4", BMI normal) Mary is getting married in five months and she wants to be looking her absolute best for the big day. She is already in good shape but would like to decrease her % body fat a little and tone up further, in particular her upper body, as this is the part that will be on show in her wedding dress. She also wants to make sure her new-found fitness levels, nutrition habits, and dedication last well after her honeymoon! Let's see if we can make this SMART for Mary:

- Specific – The wedding day date is set, so we have a very specific amount of time. We also have an upper body muscle group focus, so I can set specific exercises to strengthen and tone these areas. We need to look at her diet and be specific on what she is fuelling her body with, to ensure it is optimal to achieve her goal. Milestones are also set for the measurements taken which are very specific (e.g. 25% body fat, weight 60kg, waist 68cm etc...)

- Measurable – There are a number of measurements to take. Eight points on the body are taken with a tape measure (in cm). I have specific scales to measure weight, visceral fat (around the internal organs), daily calorie requirements, and % body fat. These measurements will ensure I can keep track on Mary's progress, to ensure she is heading in the right direction each month.

- Achievable – Mary is already in a good place and has the correct mindset to be able to achieve her goals. The specific milestones to hit are not unreasonable based on her starting point, and can be achieved within five months, and without being too extreme with the progress.

- Relevant – This is the most relevant and worthwhile goal a girl can have! To look and feel amazing on your wedding day!

- Time-bound – We have five months to complete this goal. There is a set deadline that we are working towards that isn't going to change. With planning, each month will bring a new milestone and progress to keep Mary engaged and feeling positive.

Summary

SMART goals provide a framework for setting goals that are specific, measurable, achievable, relevant, and time-bound. By incorporating these principles into our goal-setting process, we create a clear pathway to success, and therefore happiness. SMART goals help us define and focus on our objectives, track our progress, maintain motivation, and make efficient use of our time and resources. So, the next time you set a goal, remember to make it SMART and increase your chances of turning your dreams into reality.

Action Time

This is a written action.

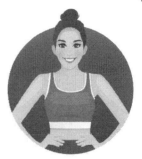

1. Using the space on the following page, have a go at writing down a SMART goal.

2. Go through the pointers in the aforementioned chapter.

3. See if you can use this exercise to stick to your chosen goal.

My example: My goal is to be able to bicep-curl 12kg dumbbells.

S – I have been specific with the exact weight, piece of equipment, and exercise.

M – I can measure if I am able to perform this move and if I can work up to it from where I can curl at the moment.

A – I curl 8kg dumbbells at the moment, so already have a level of ability, so should be able to increase this to 12kg.

R – I am used to lifting heavy weights for my job, so to be able to do this will be relevant to my job and my personal pride.

T – I would like to be able to do this within two months. I will check in at one month as well to see if I am progressing quickly enough to meet my deadline.

LIVE HAPPY

Lady Luck or hard graft?

"The harder I work, the luckier I get."

Gary Player

Retired South African multi-award-winning Champion golfer

There has always been a debate whether creating happiness is a matter of pure luck or if it requires hard work and effort. Being in the right place at the right time with positive opportunities at work, meeting the person you are destined to marry at a random party, being a naturally positive person where things just seem to go well – are these Lady Luck or due to a sequence of hard work to get to that point? In this chapter, we will explore both perspectives, examining how luck and hard work can influence your ability to find happiness.

The role of luck in happiness

Luck, often seen as a slightly mysterious force, can play a significant role in a person's happiness. How is it that some individuals seem to stumble upon happiness effortlessly, while others struggle to find it despite their best efforts. My sister, for example, has been playing the National Lottery for over 15 years and, despite her best efforts and hardest positive thinking, she is still not a jackpot winner!! Damn it!! She is not happy about this... !

Here are a few factors that highlight the role of luck in the pursuit of happiness:

Circumstances: The circumstances we are born into, such as the country, economic status, and family, greatly shape our experiences and opportunities. Those who are fortunate enough to be born in prosperous countries with loving and supportive families may find happiness more easily.

To give you an example, here are the top 10 happiest countries, listed in The World Happiness Report, published by the Sustainable Development Solutions Network, an initiative of the United Nations. The report defines happiness by using the following variables: real GDP per capita, social support, healthy life expectancy, freedom to make life choices, generosity, and perceptions of corruption.

1. Finland

2. Denmark

3. Iceland

4. Israel

5. Netherlands

6. Sweden

7. Norway

8. Switzerland

9. Luxembourg

10. New Zealand

(United Kingdom is 19th, Afghanistan is 137th)

You cannot help being born in Afghanistan but your circumstances will not help your happiness levels – you are likely to be fighting an uphill battle.

Chance encounters: Sometimes, happiness may be the result of chance encounters or unexpected events. Meeting someone who becomes a lifelong partner, stumbling upon a fulfilling career, or even getting a stroke of luck in financial matters can significantly impact one's happiness.

I can pinpoint the exact moment that my life took a turn from a business perspective – but I wouldn't know it until three years later! In the summer of 2014, my family were invited to a BBQ with friends that we had known for many years. One of the other guests, Louise, was their personal trainer. She was a good friend of theirs and had helped them with their fitness journeys. We got chatting and I asked if she could organise a group class for my team at work, as she lived very close to where our office was based. They were a roaring success and we continued these classes for three years, even when we moved offices. Due to the exposure and learnings of Louise and to these classes, I then set up my own company Work In Your Work Out Ltd, which eventually became Live Happy.

Genetic predisposition: Research suggests that a person's genetic makeup can influence their disposition towards happiness. Some individuals may naturally possess a more optimistic outlook, making it easier for them to experience happiness without extensively working for it. This is covered in more detail later.

The importance of hard work in happiness

While an element of luck can offer fortuitous opportunities, true and lasting happiness often requires persistent effort and hard work. Here are a few reasons why:

Personal growth and fulfilment: Engaging in meaningful work, pursuing passions, and investing time in nurturing relationships can lead to personal growth and fulfilment. These endeavours require dedication and effort, contributing significantly to an individual's sense of happiness.

Resilience and adaptability: Life is full of ups and downs, and cultivating resilience and adaptability is crucial in finding happiness. Cultivating these qualities requires effort and the willingness to work through challenges, ultimately leading to greater happiness and satisfaction.

Developing positive habits: As stated in the 'Exploring habits and addictions' chapter, research suggests that happiness is closely tied to habits and mindset. By actively adopting positive habits such as practising gratitude, maintaining physical and mental well-being, and seeking personal growth, individuals can increase their chances of finding happiness.

The interplay between luck and hard work

"Success = talent + luck
Great success = a little more talent + a lot of luck!"

Daniel Kahneman
Author of *Thinking Fast and Slow*

Whilst luck and hard work are often perceived as opposing forces, they are not mutually exclusive. In reality, they often interact with and influence each other in the pursuit of happiness.

Maximising opportunities: Luck can present unexpected opportunities, but seizing those opportunities requires the readiness to work hard. By cultivating a proactive mindset and putting in the effort to capitalise on fortunate circumstances, individuals can increase their chances of achieving happiness.

Overcoming adversity: Life is full of challenges, and resilience is crucial in overcoming them. Sometimes, it is luck that allows individuals to bounce back from difficult situations. However, hard work and perseverance often play a fundamental role in transforming setbacks into growth opportunities, ultimately leading to greater happiness.

Summary

In the quest for happiness, both luck and hard work play vital roles. While, if you can find it, luck can provide a head start or fortuitous opportunities, long-term happiness is often built on the foundations of hard work, personal growth, and resilience. By embracing both a bit of luck and mainly hard work, individuals can navigate their path towards happiness with a balanced and holistic approach.

Action Time

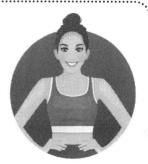

This is a written action.

1. Using the space on the following page, write down the last time you experienced good fortune.

2. Next, write down the exact circumstances.

3. Decide if you think it was 100% luck or were there circumstances leading up to the good fortune that were cultivated from hard work and perseverance?

My example: The last piece of 'luck' I had was a client thinking of me and asking if I needed anything from their work gym, as the company was refurbishing. It was brilliant timing as I was looking to get some new pieces for one of my gyms! Brilliant luck, or continuous hard work in nurturing a client relationship?

1D – HAPPINESS OVER TIME

Happiness over time

"The upside of getting older: As people age, they tend to become happier and more satisfied with their lives. Middle-aged people are the least happy, have the lowest levels of life satisfaction and the highest levels of anxiety." (The Happiness Project)

One thing that is certain in life, is that things change! We grow and age, the world around us changes; technology, advances in science, views and opinions, and people come and go in our lives. We can choose to embrace this change, or we can try to fight against it. Fight and you will always lose!

When researching the concept of whether happiness changes over time, I looked to my pursuit of happiness over my life so far and I would suggest it's a similar tale to many others. As a young child, I looked to please my parents and teachers; winning prizes and getting good results seemingly brought me happiness. As a teenager, I looked to seek additional happiness by going out with friends, owning the latest fashion trends, and being allowed the responsibility of more freedom. As a young adult with the financial ability to select my own options, I found happiness in owning a house, going on holidays that I chose, and having full independence.

Once children arrived, happiness then took a very different turn. It was much less about my own happiness and almost entirely about my children's. Now my children are no longer babies, this pursuit of happiness has changed once more. And how will it evolve when I get older still?

A comprehensive study from the Happiness Research Institute tackles an extremely important point about our ageing population. As a nation, we need to have a better plan to ensure everyone, at any age, has the chance for happiness. Matt Weiking, CEO of the Happiness Research Institute states that, *"We must ensure that longer lives also mean better lives."* This statement makes me think about my happiness in the future.

Making a very large assumption I am just over halfway through my life, what would I like to achieve that I haven't done already? What would make me truly happy? The last chapter in this section took me quite a while to compose, but it summarises my answer to this question...

From looking inward, I conclude that the concept of happiness is neither static nor universal; it transforms and adapts as we progress through different stages of life. However, several factors play a role in shaping the evolution of our pursuit of happiness. These factors include:

Life transitions: Milestones such as graduation, getting married, becoming parents, or retiring, can significantly affect our priorities, leading to shifts in our pursuit of happiness. These transitions prompt us to reassess our values and re-evaluate what truly matters.

Personal growth and wisdom: As we accumulate life experiences, learn from successes and failures, and grow emotionally and intellectually, our understanding of happiness becomes more nuanced. We begin to prioritise personal growth, self-awareness, and deep connections that contribute to a sense of fulfilment.

Changing social and cultural context: Socioeconomic changes, cultural shifts, and evolving societal expectations can influence our collective understanding of happiness and shape our personal pursuits. Cultural norms and values that emphasise community, altruism, and balance can transform our perspective on what happiness means.

Shifting perspectives on well-being: Research in positive psychology has shed light on the importance of overall well-being, which encompasses physical, mental, and social factors. As we recognise the interplay between these elements, our pursuit of happiness becomes more holistic, focusing on maintaining a healthy and balanced lifestyle.

Summary

The pursuit of happiness is not a static endeavour; it evolves alongside our growth and life experiences. As we progress through various stages of life, our priorities, values, and definitions of happiness change. Recognising this evolution empowers us to adapt and find fulfilment in new ways, embracing personal growth, meaningful connections, and a sense of purpose. By understanding how our pursuit of happiness changes over time, we can align our efforts and intentions with our current stage in life, leading to a more fulfilled and satisfying existence.

Action Time

This is a written action.

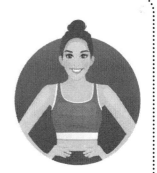

1. Using the space on the following page, write down three things that have happened in the past that made you very happy at the time.

2. Please read the chapter '50 things before I'm 50', complete the task, then come back to this page.

3. Now compare your answers to point 1 with your answers to the other chapter. Has the list of things that make you happy changed, or are you still seeking happiness in the same tasks as when you were younger?

My examples:

Younger – When I was younger, the things that made me happy were: winning a gymnastics competition, having a fun summer holiday with my family, and riding my Muddy Fox bike at the weekend.

Now – Going on a fun summer holiday is definitely still on my list. I also still love completing challenges and winning medals, but looking at my list of 50 things, they are more focused on luxury experiences that I get to do without my children!!

Parenthood

Parenthood is a transformative journey that is usually filled with incredible moments of joy, love, and fulfilment. However, it is also important to acknowledge that it comes with its fair share of challenges and quite a few moments of unhappiness. In this chapter, I explore the complex nature of finding happiness through having children, understanding the hard work involved, and how embracing both the joys and the struggles can lead to profound fulfilment.

I have written this from the perspective of being a parent. I have two young teenage sons and am genuinely finding this the most challenging time of my life so far. Although being a parent can bring you happiness and joy, it can also be a very huge source of stress and difficulty.

The joys of parenthood

Becoming a parent brings an enormous sense of purpose. The love for your child is unlike any other – it is completely unconditional and your children have a strong power over you that is extremely difficult to explain rationally. Witnessing their milestones, experiencing their first giggles, and sharing in their accomplishments, are moments that amplify happiness and create lasting memories. Parenthood allows you to discover a depth of love and joy that is uniquely tied to the growth and well-being of your children.

Embracing the challenges

However, I caveat this with the fact that parenting is not without its challenges. Sleepless nights, juggling responsibilities, and the constant worry for your child's well-being can bring lots of moments of stress and unhappiness. It is important to acknowledge that these challenges are a natural part of parenthood and that it is OK to feel completely overwhelmed at times. By embracing and working through these difficulties, we grow as individuals and develop resilience, patience, and adaptability. The path to happiness through parenthood lies in understanding that the challenges are part of the journey, and that we can learn and grow alongside our children. And I hate to say this, but sometimes a large glass of wine also helps!!

"Most people would say their children are one of the greatest source of happiness. However, research suggests the opposite. Why do we have an intuition that is entirely at odds with the data? Here are the researchers answers:

1. *People are prepared to pay a lot for things they love, and they tend to love the more they had to pay for it. Raising children is hard work, and you pay for them in every way, not only in the form of money but also in blood, sweat, tears, and hair.*

2. *A child's basic needs are very demanding. This crowds out other sources of pleasure in the parents' life with the child becoming a major source of happy moments.*

3. *People mainly remember episodes by their highest peaks and their final moments. Even if you spent an entire day mostly saying to your child; 'Don't do this, not now, don't hit your sister, I already told you no, no I'm not buying it...' all the hassle may get blanked out by just a single 'Dad, I love you', 'Mum, you are the best mum in the world."*

(The Happiness Project)

The reward of hard work

Parenthood requires dedication, sacrifice, and hard work. The effort put into raising children can be exhausting, demanding, and relentless. But remember that the milestones achieved, the values instilled, and the bond forged with your children are the result of your commitment and love. The satisfaction that comes from seeing your child grow into a caring, responsible, and successful individual cannot be understated. The lessons we learn from the hard work of parenting contribute to our personal growth and fulfilment.

To give you a few examples from my experience so far: I'm that mum standing on the side of the football pitch jumping up and down shouting, "Well done, baby!" to my teenage son when he scores a goal – utterly embarrassing to my child, but the pride swelling over when either of them does anything at all that's positive; I just can't help myself! I'm that mum weeping with joy when they receive an award at school (for one of them, it was pretty rare so made it even more special when he did!). I'm also that mum driving around the UK each weekend, supporting them with their chosen hobbies and using almost all of my earnings on paying for these very expensive sports. I'm exhausted all the time due to the family and work schedule we have each week, but that's just what you do! I spend a large amount of time just hoping that my two little boys grow up to be kind, useful members of society, able to keep their mother in the manner in which she is accustomed!!

Finding balance and self-care

A very important yet often forgotten point is that parenthood is not solely about the happiness of your children, but also should include your personal happiness and well-being. It is essential to find balance within the demands of parenting and prioritise self-care. Taking time for yourself, pursuing your interests, and maintaining a strong support system are crucial for maintaining your own happiness. By nurturing yourself, you create a positive environment for both you and your children, ensuring a more fulfilling parenting experience.

My child-coping mechanism to get through the year in one piece is to book a mini break with my sister once a year – over the years, we have been to Malta, Tenerife, and Ibiza. This is my one chance to have a proper break – not being someone's mum, but to spend some quality time with my wonderful sister, without the kids interrupting every conversation we have. It feels indulgent and does heavily rely on my husband being able to cope for a few days without my help, but it is something that I look forward to all year and keeps me sane!

Summary

Parenthood is a journey that encompasses both incredible joy and moments of unhappiness. Understanding the complexities and embracing the challenges allows us to find profound happiness. The love, growth, and fulfilment that come from raising children outweigh the hardships (sometimes only just!). By accepting the difficulties, putting in the necessary work, and prioritising self-care, we can navigate the ups and downs of parenthood and experience the immense happiness that comes from watching our children flourish and being an integral part of their lives.

Action Time

This is a written action.

There will be times when your children drive you completely bonkers and you cannot think about how to not feel very annoyed and/or terribly sad.

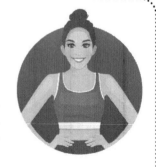

When this happens, please use the space below to write down either the last time your child/children did something that made you extremely proud of them, or when you last had a fun time with them.

1. Write down how this made you feel, and how your words and actions made them feel.

2. When you find yourself feeling unhappy with them, come back to this page and remember your words.

My example: When my eldest child won his first karting trophy, I remember his proud, happy, little face when he was presented with it. Children are designed to make their parents think they are super cute and amazing, even if they can sometimes be little monsters – they are very clever!!

Viewing life like a child

Sometimes (definitely not all the time!) I am very jealous of my children! Apart from the fact they have boundless energy and the weight of the world hasn't fallen on their shoulders yet (they are too young for exams or mortgages!), they can find pure, unadulterated joy and happiness in the simplest of things. Finding a frog in the garden and watching it with fascination, screaming with utter joy at winning an online game with their friends, finding something on their iPad so funny that they simply cannot stop laughing, sitting with our dog stroking his head, so comfortable and warm. And they are 'tweenagers' now – it was even more innocent and pure when they were tiny. If only we could harness this utter happiness at the simple things. I think we may be able to...

While the pursuit of happiness is universal, understanding the science behind why children can harness this state more easily is a fascinating exploration. In this chapter, we will delve into the factors contributing to children's ability to find joy and offer insights into how adults can recapture that childlike happiness.

The innocence advantage

Present-moment awareness: Children naturally dwell in the present moment, uninhibited by past regrets or future anxieties. This form of mindfulness allows them to fully immerse themselves in the experiences and sensations unfolding before them. By focusing their attention on the here and now, children can embrace the simplicity and wonder of the present.

Emotional expressiveness: Children freely express their emotions, unrestrained by societal norms or fear of judgement. Their ability to vividly exhibit and process emotions enhances their capacity for genuine happiness. By fully embracing and expressing their feelings, children experience the release and joy that comes with emotional authenticity.

Curiosity and wonder

Sense of discovery: Children possess an insatiable curiosity that drives them to explore and understand the world around them. This thirst for knowledge and discovery enhances their overall happiness as they continuously encounter new experiences and learn from them. By adopting a mindset of continuous learning and exploration, adults can tap into the same sense of wonder and excitement.

Ability to find joy in the simplest things: Children find immense joy in even the smallest and simplest of things, whether it's chasing a butterfly, blowing bubbles, or laughing uncontrollably. Their ability to appreciate the little pleasures in life allows them to experience happiness more readily. As adults, reconnecting with this appreciation can open up new avenues of happiness.

Resilience and adaptability

Letting go of expectations: Children approach life with fewer preconceived notions and expectations. They embrace experiences as they come, without judgements or comparisons. This openness and willingness to adapt contribute to their ability to find happiness in various situations. By releasing attachment to certain outcomes, adults can enhance their own resilience and allow happiness to emerge more naturally.

Embracing play and creativity: Playfulness is a key characteristic of childhood, facilitating the exploration of imaginative, creative, and carefree experiences. Engaging in playful activities allows children to tap into their innate happiness. Adults who reintroduce playfulness into their lives can break free from the constraints of adulthood, leading to increased joy and happiness.

Nurturing childlike happiness

I was pleasantly surprised to read the findings of Dr Lara Aknin who, with UBC colleagues Professors Kiley Hamlin and Elizabeth Dunn, studied young children and their happiness:

"People tend to assume that toddlers are naturally selfish ... these findings show that children are actually happier giving than receiving. What's most exciting about these findings is that children are happiest when giving their own treats away ... Forfeiting their own valuable resources for the benefit of others, makes them happier than giving away just any treat." (Aknin et al, 2012)

Their studies also concluded that even from a very young age, the act of helping or being kind to someone else is deeply woven into our nature. It can also answer the long-standing question of why we like to help others, including people we have just met. It gives us positive feelings of happiness that we enjoy.

Cultivating gratitude: Encouraging gratitude practice helps adults focus on the positive aspects of their lives. By consciously recognising and appreciating the blessings they have, adults can foster a childlike sense of wonder and contentment.

Mindfulness and present-moment awareness: Practicing mindfulness can help adults to slow down, observe their surroundings, and savour the present moment. By reconnecting with the present, they can rekindle the same awe and appreciation that children naturally possess.

Embracing play and creativity: Incorporating playfulness and creativity into daily life helps unlock the inner child. Engaging in activities that bring joy and spontaneity can reintroduce a sense of play and reignite the happiness that accompanies it. Next time you have a moment, get some paper and crayons out and just draw what comes to your mind – you might be quite surprised how creative you can get and that it's quite relaxing to scribble like you used to when you were young.

Summary

While adulthood brings its own set of challenges and responsibilities, adults can learn valuable lessons from children about effortlessly harnessing pure happiness. By embodying childlike qualities such as curiosity, wonder, resilience, and playfulness, adults can rediscover the joy that accompanies the simple pleasures of life. By understanding the science behind children's happiness, we can apply these principles to our own lives, nurturing a state of happiness that is authentic, genuine, and enduring.

Action Time

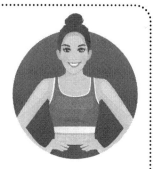

This is a written action.

1. Using the space on the following page, write down two things that you did when you were younger that epitomised happiness for you.

2. Now write down the memories this invokes for you and if this reminds you of a certain place, person, smell, or feeling.

My examples:

The feeling of moving back and forth on a swing; the sun on my face and a slight breeze as I move gently back and forth. This reminds me of the school summer holidays at home with my friend Sarah, in the strawberry fields near our houses.

Playing a classic, simple board game such as Connect4 or Snakes & Ladders – this is the feeling of gaining on my opponent, laughing, and innocent fun – no digital tech!

Look up and experience life, don't let it pass you by

I don't often need to commute into London so for me it is a bit more of a novelty. However, recently, I had to attend a conference, so I caught the early morning train. The platform was packed to the rafters with bored, tired, slightly impatient commuters.

I know it is tedious waiting for anything, but without exception, every single person standing on that platform was bent over their phone, either typing or watching something! I was looking at a sea of poor posture! The first thing I thought was that it is no wonder that I am dealing with clients' back and neck issues and discomfort all the time!

I was also looking at a set of people that were letting hours pass them by without noticing anything at all – not allowing themselves to add anything to their lives that morning. In fact, probably most mornings for years.

In today's digital age, our lives seem inseparable from our smartphones, tablets, and laptops. While technology has undoubtedly brought many conveniences and benefits, it's important to recognise the value of looking up from our screens and fully experiencing the world around us. In this chapter, we will explore the significance of disconnecting from digital devices and reconnecting with our physical environment to enrich our lives and create meaningful experiences.

The lost art of presence

In our constant pursuit of virtual connections and digital engagements, we often overlook the beauty and richness of the present moment. Absorbed in our screens, we miss out on the sights, sounds, and interactions that can bring us joy and fulfilment. By consciously choosing to look up from our phones and engage with the world, we can cultivate a sense of presence that allows us to fully experience life.

Appreciating the surroundings

Beauty in the mundane: When we take the time to observe and appreciate our surroundings, we discover beauty in the ordinary. Whether it's the play of light and shadow on a city street, or the intricate details of nature, the world around us is teeming with wonders waiting to be noticed. I beg you – on your next commute, look up and look around you. What can you see, smell, observe, learn? People watching is absolutely fascinating!

Fostering connections: Human connections are paramount to our well-being. By putting away our devices and engaging with others, we can build stronger relationships, deepen our understanding, and develop empathy. Engaging in face-to-face conversations fosters a sense of inclusion, belonging, and emotional fulfilment.

Being present for personal growth

Mindfulness and stress reduction: Being present and focusing on the present moment is at the heart of mindfulness practices. Taking a break from our screens and being fully engaged with our surroundings can help reduce stress levels, increase self-awareness, and improve overall mental well-being.

Sparking creativity: Our surroundings often hold inspiration for our creative endeavours. By observing and interacting with the environment, we expose ourselves to new ideas, perspectives, and experiences that can fuel our imagination and spark innovative thinking.

Cultivating gratitude: When we disconnect from our screens and appreciate the world around us, we become more attuned to the simple pleasures and everyday blessings that we often take for granted. This shift in perspective fosters a sense of gratitude, which has been linked to higher levels of happiness and life satisfaction.

Creating healthy digital habits

Set boundaries: Establish specific times and places where you disconnect from screens and commit to being fully present. Designate 'tech-free zones' or 'tech-free hours' to encourage a healthier balance between online and offline experiences.

Practice mindful screen use: When using digital devices, be intentional about how you spend your time. Regularly assess whether your screen time aligns with your values, goals, and overall well-being. Consider engaging in activities that promote learning, creativity, or meaningful connections.

Engage in outdoor activities: Spending time in nature can be both rejuvenating and inspiring. Seek opportunities to immerse yourself in outdoor activities, such as hiking, gardening, or simply taking a stroll in the park. These experiences can reconnect you with the natural world and provide a necessary break from the digital realm.

Although there is a danger I am going to sound like an old, ranting person, I have also observed the habits of the average teenager. Having two myself, teaching teenage students and living near a number of schools and a college, it is extremely obvious that teenagers are definitely not looking up from their phones and experiencing the joys of life around them. Some are even walking next to each other and instead of looking up and talking, they are texting responses to the person next to them!

If you are going to spend a proportion of your life doing the same thing, why not try to find happiness in it? Use your commute in a productive way that is not going to damage your neck and back muscles. Use your walk to school talking and enjoying the company of your friends and looking around at your neighbourhood.

Summary

In a world consumed by screens, it is crucial to remember the importance of looking up from our phones and experiencing life first hand. By disconnecting from digital devices and engaging with our surroundings, we can cultivate a sense of presence, foster deeper connections, experience personal growth, and embrace the beauty and wonders of the world. Let us not merely exist in a virtual world but actively participate in the journey of life, creating meaningful moments and lasting memories.

Action Time

This is a practical action.

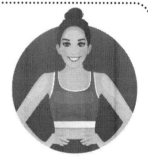

1. When you are on your next commute (it might even be right now as you are reading this book!), subtly observe two people sitting closest to you.

2. Let your imagination run free and make up a story to yourself about who they are, what they do, where they live. Not only is it a great way to pass the time, it's creatively stimulating and can be very amusing.

My example: I am sitting opposite a man on the train. He has plain, dark clothing on, his hood is up, and he is texting. He is actually a spy for the British government and is on a special mission to save the country. He has just been texted his next mission by 'M' and is on his way to London to meet with his colleague, pick up his Aston Martin, and drive to the South of France to spy on an international criminal... ☺

50 things before I'm 50

Something I have found particularly useful is composing a list. It is surprising how much I have enjoyed composing this as it is Not Just Any List! It is 50 things I would like to achieve before the age of 50. At the time of writing, I have seven years left to complete it...

This exercise encourages you to clarify and prioritise what activities and purchases will make you happy, and how you are going to use your finances wisely. They don't all have to be massive and overly expensive – in fact, unless you have a huge pot of money, then they can't all be massive!

To help inspire you, here's my list, in no particular order. I have marked the ones I have already managed to achieve – if you are reading this and think you may be able to help me out with any I haven't done yet, please drop me a line! Very happy to chat!

1.   Write a book and have it published – DONE

2.   Read a novel in one day (have the time to) – DONE

3.   Re-visit Barbados – my most favourite place

4.   Visit Dubai

5.   Visit Japan

6.   Experience clubbing in Ibiza – DONE

7.   Enjoy a top-end cruise/yacht charter

8.   Complete a triathlon (even if it's not a full one) – DONE

9.   Purchase the remaining third of my rings (the eternity ring that sits with my wedding and engagement rings)

10. Gain a counselling qualification – DONE

11. Test-drive a supercar

12. Find the perfect online gluten-free afternoon tea

13. Own an expensive pair of prescription sunglasses (Prada PR32PS Heritage) – DONE

14. Stay in a cute cottage in Cornwall

15. Create something on a pottery wheel

16. Act in, or be an extra in, a film

17. Have an all-day shopping trip (without my kids!)

18. Obtain a massage qualification

19. Have a 'post-aged 40' photo taken of myself that I'm really proud of (and that I'm allowed to publish)

20. Get a tattoo – DONE

21. Travel to the airport, book a flight to anywhere, and go for the weekend!

22. Swim in crystal clear natural water

23. Spend the whole day watching films in my PJs (and not be forced to because I'm ill!)

24. Have a full pampering day (hair, nails, massage, waxing, etc...) – DONE

25. Spend a whole month on holiday

26. Travel on a luxury train

27. Stay in a chalet in the snow

28. Watch a movie at the London IMAX

29. Have a dress tailor-made for me – DONE

30. Cruise around the Croatian islands

31. Become mortgage free!

32. Enjoy a drink in 10 of the most famous hotels in London: The Landmark, Claridge's, Shangri-La The Shard, The Ritz, The Langham, The Savoy, The Sheraton Grand London Park Lane, The Dorchester, Brown's Hotel, The Four Seasons Hotel.

33. Watch the sunrise and sunset in one day

34. Be on a radio show (either as the presenter or the interviewee)

35. Feel like a princess for a weekend and stay in a castle

36. Experience a professional make-up session

37. Have a personal shopping session

38. Create a piece of jewellery

39. Learn how to say "Thank you" in 10 different languages

40. Ride on a tandem bike

41. Eat only veggie for a month – DONE

42. Own a beautiful set of underwear

43. Experience a proper, snowy White Christmas

44. Experience all the 'playing cards of Henley'. (Henley town have produced a deck of 52 cards that have the top places to

visit or things to do in the town. As I live there, I thought it important and interesting to complete the list!)

45. Take a bike tour of Amsterdam – DONE

46. Re-read all the *Harry Potter* books

47. Go whale and dolphin watching – DONE

48. Create a cross stitch cushion – DONE

49. Bathe in a natural hot spring

50. Have one of my social media posts/blog go viral

I wasn't that surprised to notice that a large proportion of my list was travel related! Even from a very young age, annual holidays are remembered and cherished – they are special, different, exciting, memorable, and usually very positive moments in life that can capture the feeling of happiness. Very few of my 50 things are products that are purchased, they are much more 'experience' related. A few are also achievement and learning/development related. As humans, we seek self-improvement and grow by adding to our current skill set. It is very important for our mental health and well-being.

I will be focusing a chunk of my energy and finances on managing to achieve my full list in the coming years. Updates are available on my social media channels. You will know that I have achieved the first one, as you are reading it!!

Action time

This is a written action.

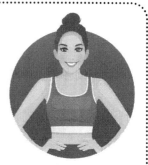

1.   Using the space on the following page, write a list of what you would like to achieve in life that will make you happy, even if it's not as many as the decade you are in currently.

2.   Start with 10 things and build on it.

3.   Take your time, come back to it frequently, and evaluate whether this is a true ambition or just a passing whim.

4.   Publish your list on social media so your friends and family can see it – this will hold you more accountable to achieving it!

My example: In my list, I thought about a mix of geographical locations I would like to visit, activities and experiences I would like to try, possessions I would like to own, and challenges I would like to overcome. Then I posted it on Instagram, LinkedIn and Facebook, created a blog about it ,and verbally told all my friends, family and clients. It's also in black and white in this book! Got to do it all now!! ☺

MOVE

As previously stated, exercise, movement, and remaining healthy are crucial to maintaining happiness. In this section of the book, I delve into further detail as to why we should build exercise into our weekly routines, the art of enjoying the exercise you choose to do, and remaining motivated. I also include a simple set of relaxation techniques and some exercise programme ideas for when you have access to gym equipment and for when you don't. Use this section of the book to gain some exercise inspiration and some knowledge about the workings of your body.

Your health, physical, and mental well-being are everything. A great job and lovely things around you mean nothing if you don't have your health. Look after your body and it will thank you in the long term. Seek help to do this as well – surround yourself with positive people and tools that help you.

'Let's get physical...'
Why should humans exercise?

Getting all hormonal

"Health and Happiness: Not everyone who is healthy is happy. And not everyone who is sick is miserable. But those who are happy more often are less sick and live longer. Happiness protects you against heart attacks, autoimmune disorders, diabetes, cancer, and the opposite of happiness; depression." (The Happiness Project)

Humans are so clever! When we do something that is good for us, our body thanks us. In the short term, when we exercise, our body releases wonderful, natural chemicals called endorphins – hormones that act as natural painkillers and create a mini feeling of euphoria. Endorphins also help to reduce stress and anxiety levels. Exercise also increases the production of serotonin, a neurotransmitter known to regulate mood, appetite, and sleep. No one believes this when they first start exercising, but I promise you, it will happen! I know the effort of getting on the treadmill is hard, but when you have finished, you will feel those hormones pulsating through your body. You will think, "Actually, that was worth it! I feel more positive now!" Clever us!

Exercise is a natural energy power boost button

If you find yourself feeling sluggish, tired, or low on energy, exercise can help boost your energy levels naturally – no need for six cups of coffee each morning! Exercise increases blood flow, ensuring that your organs and muscles are getting the necessary nutrients and oxygen. Additionally, exercise increases stamina, so you can tackle daily activities with less exertion. The caveat that I would add to this is if this really isn't working and you are constantly shattered, you could have low iron levels or a medical issue, such as an underactive thyroid. I would suggest seeing your GP as soon as possible.

Long-term benefits

There are a number of long-term benefits to regular exercise, not just the initial chemical rush! You will start to notice your body shape changing – this depends on what type of exercise you are doing and how frequently, but any kind of movement will improve muscle tone and ensure your muscles continue to improve. Body composition is the important thing here – **not** weight loss. This may sound a little controversial, but I ask people to worry less about their weight and more about their muscle/fat % ratio changing for the better. You are not trying to lose weight, you are trying to improve the way you look and feel in your own body. Weight loss is just a potential by-product. Weighing yourself is a good measure to take, but don't get obsessed with it. In fact, exercise may actually increase your weight as muscle is more dense than fat. But don't worry – what does it matter what you weigh if you are losing inches, toning up, and feeling a lot better?

Mr Motivator

You have now discovered that exercise helps you to feel better using those wonderful natural chemicals and you have started to see the longer-term benefits of exercise, but how do you stay motivated to keep going? This is part of something called the Transtheoretical Model of Behaviour Change. Your brain is going through a series of decisions on whether to carry on or give yourself a reason to stop. However, my experience working with clients over many years is that when it comes to exercise and getting results, consistency is key. Finding an exercise routine that feels enjoyable, challenging, and rewarding is essential. This is likely to change over time as well. Setting a specific workout schedule and timing, or working out with a friend, can really help hold you accountable and keep you motivated. I personally much prefer working out with someone else, ideally someone stronger or faster than me to keep me on my toes!!

What to choose?

There are countless ways to get moving and incorporate exercise into your daily routine. Aerobic exercise, also known as cardio, elevates the heart rate, burns calories, and strengthens the cardiovascular system. Strength training, such as weightlifting, can help build muscle mass, increase bone density, and burn calories. Yoga offers a mix of breath work, stretching, and strength training that is known for its calming effects on the mind and body. And there is everything in between!

Summary

Incorporating exercise into your daily routine has numerous mental, physical, and emotional benefits. By releasing endorphins, improving moods, boosting energy, and decreasing stress levels, regular exercise can help you to feel a lot happier now and later in your life.

Embrace your inner gym bunny

Physical exercise is a crucial component of a healthy lifestyle, but for many, the idea of hitting the gym or going for a run can be a nightmare. The noisy free-weights section, full of intimidating biceps! People on the running machines who look like they can easily run a marathon without breaking a sweat! The personal trainers who either pester you to sign up to 10 sessions with them, or who hog all of the machines for their clients! It doesn't have to be this way though – honestly! With the right mindset and a few simple strategies, you can turn being at the gym into a fun and fulfilling experience. In this chapter, we will explore the art of enjoying exercise and provide you with some top tips to make your fitness journey more pleasurable.

Find activities you love

The key to enjoying exercise is finding activities that bring you genuine pleasure. Experiment with various types of workouts such as dancing, hiking, swimming, team sports, or yoga. Embrace the idea that there is no one-size-fits-all approach to fitness. Once you discover activities you genuinely enjoy, exercising will no longer feel like a burden.

Set realistic goals

Setting achievable goals is essential for sustained enjoyment of exercise. Focus on your personal progress rather than comparing yourself to others. Whether it's running a certain distance, increasing your strength, or improving flexibility, break your goals down into smaller milestones. Celebrate each achievement along the way, and remember that progress takes time.

Make it social

Exercising with friends or joining a group class can turn your fitness routine into a social occasion. The support and camaraderie fostered through shared physical activity can make exercising more enjoyable. Schedule regular group workouts or organise friendly competitions to add an element of fun and motivation to your exercise regime.

Incorporate variety

Repetitive workouts can feel monotonous and lead to boredom. Keep things exciting and enjoyable by incorporating variety into your exercise routine. Try different types of workouts, explore new trails, or experiment with various fitness classes. Mixing things up will keep you engaged and prevent staleness.

Focus on the journey, not just the outcome

Sometimes, we become too fixated on achieving specific results and forget to enjoy the process. Embrace the journey of exercise, appreciating the physical sensations, and the mental clarity it brings. Shift your mindset from solely focusing on desired outcomes to embracing the holistic benefits of movement, such as increased energy levels, stress relief, and improved overall well-being.

Find a workout buddy

Exercising with a partner or a supportive friend can make workouts more enjoyable. A workout buddy can provide motivation, hold you accountable, and turn exercise into a bonding experience. Choose someone who shares your fitness goals and interests, and together, you can make your workouts more engaging and fun.

Personalise your routine

Tailor your exercise routine to suit your preferences and interests. If you enjoy being outdoors, take advantage of the natural scenery by going for hikes or biking. If you're a music lover, create energising playlists to accompany your workouts. Personalising your routine adds extra motivation and makes exercise feel more enjoyable and reflective of your unique personality.

Summary

Embracing the art of enjoying exercise involves finding activities you love, setting realistic goals, incorporating variety, and making it a social experience. Remember to focus on the journey rather than just the outcome and personalise your routine to reflect your interests and preferences. By applying these top tips, you can transform exercise from a daunting or boring chore into a source of ongoing happiness and fulfilment, making it an integral part of your daily routine.

Staying motivated

As mentioned earlier, you start your fitness journey all pumped and ready to change the world, but then boredom sets in, it all becomes a bit hard, and trips to the gym become less frequent, then non-existent. If consistency is key but you are trying to keep it interesting, how is it best to stay motivated to carry on your fitness journey?

When it comes to maintaining a fit and healthy lifestyle, motivation plays a crucial role. However, staying motivated to exercise can be a challenge for many individuals. In this chapter, we will explore various strategies to help you stay motivated, stay consistent, and achieve your fitness goals.

Setting clear and realistic goals

One of the key components of maintaining motivation is setting clear and realistic goals. Start by defining your fitness objectives, whether it's running a certain distance, losing a specific amount of weight, or increasing your strength and endurance. Break these larger goals down into smaller milestones, allowing you to celebrate achievements along the way. Setting realistic goals that align with your abilities and lifestyle will help you stay motivated by providing a sense of accomplishment and progress.

Creating a positive environment

Your environment significantly influences your motivation levels. To stay motivated, create a positive and supportive environment conducive to exercise and healthy habits.

Surround yourself with like-minded, motivated individuals: Identify exercise partners or join fitness communities that share similar goals. This will encourage accountability, collaboration, and support.

Set up an inspiring workout space: Whether you exercise at home or in a gym, personalise your environment with motivational quotes, visuals, or uplifting music. A visually appealing and motivating space can help maintain focus and drive during your workouts.

Building a consistent routine

I can't tell you how many times I say this to my clients, but consistency is vital in maintaining motivation over the long term. Establishing a routine helps make exercise a habit, ingraining it into your lifestyle.

Schedule your workouts: Treat exercise as an important appointment in your calendar. Set specific days and times for your workouts, making them non-negotiable commitments.

Start with small, manageable steps: Begin with a realistic exercise frequency and duration that you can comfortably maintain. Gradually increase the intensity and duration of your workouts as your fitness level improves.

Finding intrinsic motivators

While external motivators (such as rewards or recognition) can provide short-term boosts, finding intrinsic motivators will keep your exercise routine sustainable and enjoyable.

Discover activities you genuinely enjoy: Experiment with different forms of exercise until you find activities that align with your interests, abilities, and goals. Whether it's dancing, hiking, swimming, or weightlifting, engaging in activities you genuinely enjoy naturally fuels motivation.

Focus on the holistic benefits: Look beyond physical results. Remind yourself of the mental, emotional, and long-term health benefits of exercise, such as increased energy, reduced stress, improved mood, and better overall well-being.

Embracing accountability and tracking progress

Accountability and progress tracking provide additional motivation by showcasing your achievements and holding yourself responsible.

Share your goals: Vocalise your fitness objectives to a supportive friend, family member, or trainer. Regularly updating them on your progress creates a sense of accountability and encouragement. There is nothing quite like posting to all your friends and contacts on your social media channels that you are going to take part in a triathlon! Now you've committed!!

Keep a workout log or use fitness apps: Track your workouts, noting the exercises performed, duration, intensity, and any improvements. Reviewing your progress helps maintain motivation by visualising how far you've come and setting new targets. My favourite tracker apps are MyFitnessPal and Nutracheck Calorie Counter. And of course, a fabulous health and well-being app to definitely check out is Live Happy!

Rewarding yourself

Rewards act as an impactful motivator, especially when aligned with your fitness goals.

Set milestone rewards: Celebrate achieving significant milestones with non-food-based rewards, such as a massage, new workout attire, or a spa day. Rewarding yourself positively reinforces your efforts and keeps your motivation levels high.

Establish a personal reward system: Create a reward system that allows for small daily or weekly treats when you consistently complete your workouts. These rewards can be as simple as enjoying a favourite healthy snack, engaging in a relaxing activity, or allowing yourself guilt-free leisure time.

Summary

Maintaining motivation to exercise and keep yourself fit and healthy requires effort and conscious implementation of strategies specific to your needs. By setting achievable goals, creating a positive environment, establishing a consistent routine, finding intrinsic motivators, embracing accountability, and rewarding yourself, you can build sustainable habits that lead to a lifelong commitment to fitness, well-being, and ultimately, your ongoing happiness. Remember, motivation begins within, and with determination and perseverance, you can surpass any obstacles on your fitness journey.

What type of exercise to choose

As we know, regular exercise not only helps us stay physically fit but also has a positive impact on our mental health and therefore our happiness. There are various types of exercises, each targeting different aspects of our bodies. In this chapter, we will explore some of the most common exercise types and understand the benefits they offer. This will help you to decide the type of exercise that might be best for you, and then you can use the last chapter in this section to pick some suitable exercise plans.

Aerobic exercises

Aerobic exercises, also known as cardio exercises, focus on increasing your heart rate and improving cardiovascular health. Activities such as running, swimming, cycling, or dancing fall into this category. The benefits of aerobic exercise include:

- Improved cardiovascular fitness: Regular cardio exercises strengthen your heart and lungs, improving their efficiency.

- Weight management: Aerobic exercises burn calories, helping you maintain a healthy weight or lose excess weight.

- Enhanced mood: Engaging in cardio exercises releases endorphins, which promote feelings of happiness and reduce stress.

Strength training

Strength training exercises primarily involve working against resistance to build muscle strength and endurance. This can be achieved through weightlifting, resistance band exercises, or bodyweight exercises such as push-ups and squats. The benefits of strength training include:

- Increased muscle strength: Regular strength training helps build and tone muscles, making you stronger and more resilient.

- Metabolic boost: Strengthening your muscles through resistance training can help increase your metabolism, leading to potential long-term weight management benefits.

- Improved bone health: By stimulating the production of new bone tissue, strength training exercises can help prevent bone loss and reduce the risk of conditions like osteoporosis.

Flexibility and stretching

Flexibility exercises focus on improving joint range of motion and muscle elasticity. This includes yoga, Pilates, or dedicated stretching routines. The benefits of flexibility exercises include:

- Improved posture and balance: Stretching exercises help enhance muscle flexibility, leading to improved posture and balance.

- Reduced muscle soreness: Incorporating stretching into your exercise routine can help alleviate muscle tightness and reduce the chances of post-workout soreness.

- Injury prevention: Enhancing flexibility in muscles and joints can decrease the likelihood of injuries by allowing a wider range of motion during physical activities.

High-Intensity Interval Training (HIIT)

HIIT combines short bursts of intense exercise with recovery periods. It typically involves activities such as sprinting, burpees, or jumping jacks. The benefits of HIIT include:

- Efficient calorie burning: HIIT workouts are known for their calorie-torching capabilities, contributing to weight loss and improved fitness levels.

- Enhanced cardiovascular health: The intense intervals in HIIT training help improve cardiovascular strength and endurance.

- Time-saving: HIIT workouts often last between 15 to 30 minutes, making them a great option for individuals with limited time for exercise.

Summary

Choosing the right mix of exercises to incorporate into your fitness routine depends on your goals, preferences, and overall health condition. By exploring different exercise types like aerobic exercises, strength training, flexibility exercises, and HIIT, you can create a well-rounded routine that maximises the benefits for your body and can create a strong sense of happiness if you find a routine that really works for you. Remember to consult with a healthcare professional before starting or significantly changing your exercise regime.

Walking in Nature

One of the most popular answers in the happiness survey was going for a walk outside – whether this was on the beach, in the woods, or in the mountains. I completely agree! A good walk outside clears my head, gets me away from an electronic screen, and gets the step count up for the day. As many of my clients are mainly desk-based professionals, I strongly suggest that they take a walk every day for a minimum of 30 minutes – and it works! So, what does walking in nature do for us from psychological and physiological perspectives?

Psychological benefits

Stress reduction:

Walking in nature offers an escape from the hustle and bustle of daily life, allowing individuals to disconnect from sources of stress and find solace in the natural environment. Research suggests that spending time in nature, particularly in green spaces, can significantly reduce cortisol levels, a hormone associated with stress (Roe et al, 2013). As you take each step, surrounded by the beauty of nature, your mind can find peace and a sense of tranquillity.

Improved mental well-being:

Walking in nature has been shown to improve overall mental well-being (mind.org.uk). It promotes the release of endorphins, neurotransmitters responsible for feelings of happiness and euphoria. Nature's soothing and gentle environment can alleviate symptoms of depression, anxiety, and other mental health conditions, providing a sense of calm and renewed energy.

Enhanced cognitive function:

Nature walks have demonstrated positive effects on cognitive functions, such as attention, memory, and creativity. The mind can fully engage with the present moment, creating sharper focus and improved problem-solving abilities. Walking amidst trees and natural surroundings also stimulates our senses, triggering a cognitive boost that can enhance overall brain function.

Physiological benefits

Cardiovascular health:

Engaging in regular walks in nature can have a profound impact on cardiovascular health. Walking is a low-impact aerobic exercise that increases heart rate and circulation, promoting a healthy cardiovascular system (Murtagh et all, 2010). Studies have found that walking in nature can decrease blood pressure, lower cholesterol levels, and reduce the risk of heart disease.

Immune system boost:

Nature walks can support a robust immune system. Spending time outdoors exposes us to sunlight and fresh air, both of which provide necessary vitamins, such as vitamin D. Additionally, exposure to phytoncides – natural oils emitted by trees – has been found to enhance the activity of our natural killer (NK) cells, which play a crucial role in fighting off infections and tumours.

Improved sleep quality:

Walking in nature can also lead to better sleep quality. Exposure to natural light during the day helps regulate the body's internal clock, promoting better sleep-wake cycles. Additionally, the physical exertion of walking contributes to better sleep quality by reducing restlessness and promoting relaxation.

Summary

Walking in nature offers a multitude of psychological and physiological benefits. It provides a natural remedy for stress reduction, improves mental well-being, enhances cognitive function, promotes cardiovascular health, boosts the immune system, and improves sleep quality. By incorporating regular walks in serene natural environments into our lives, we can harness the transformative power of nature to uplift our spirits and improve our overall health and well-being. So, lace up your shoes, step outside, and let the healing magic of nature embrace you on your journey to a healthier and happier self.

Relaxation techniques for happiness

In our fast-paced and demanding lives, it is essential to prioritise relaxation and self-care to maintain optimal happiness and well-being. Engaging in relaxation techniques can help reduce stress, improve mood, and enhance overall happiness levels. They may seem a little tricky at first and can take some getting used to, but the positive benefits can be felt almost immediately, so please persevere. In this chapter, we will explore various relaxation techniques, including breathing exercises, stretching, and visualisation, and understand how they can contribute to our happiness.

Breathing techniques

Deep, intentional breathing techniques can have a profound impact on our mental and physical well-being. Some popular techniques include:

Diaphragmatic breathing: Sit or lie down in a comfortable position. Breathe in deeply through your nose, expanding your belly, and then exhale slowly through your mouth. Repeat this several times, focusing on each breath, to promote relaxation and calm.

Box breathing: Inhale deeply through your nose for a count of four, holding your breath for a count of four. Exhale slowly through your mouth for a count of four, and then hold your breath out for a count of four. Repeat this pattern for several rounds, allowing yourself to enter a more relaxed state.

4-7-8 breathing: Inhale deeply through your nose for a count of four. Hold your breath for a count of seven. Exhale slowly through your mouth for a count of eight. Repeat this cycle multiple times, feeling a sense of calm as you regulate your breathing.

Stretching and progressive muscle relaxation

Stretching exercises and progressive muscle relaxation techniques can help release tension and promote relaxation. Some techniques to try include:

Head-to-toe stretch: Start by gently stretching your neck, shoulders, arms, back, hips, legs, and feet. Focus on each muscle group, stretching it slowly and deliberately. Pay attention to any areas of tension and consciously release it as you stretch. This promotes physical relaxation and can alleviate muscle soreness.

Progressive muscle relaxation: Start by tensing a specific muscle group, such as your shoulders, for a few seconds, then release and relax the muscles completely. Move through different muscle groups, progressively working from your head down to your toes. This technique helps release physical tension and create a sense of overall relaxation.

Visualisation

Visualisation exercises involve imagining a peaceful and calming scene or situation to promote relaxation and happiness. Here's a simple visualisation technique:

Find a quiet place to sit or lie down comfortably. Close your eyes and take a few deep breaths. Visualise yourself in a serene place, such as a beach, forest, or any location that brings you joy. Engage your senses by imagining the sounds, smells, and textures of that environment. Allow yourself to immerse fully in this calming visualisation, experiencing a sense of tranquillity and happiness.

Summary

Incorporating relaxation techniques into your daily routine is vital for maintaining happiness and overall well-being. Breathing exercises, stretching, and visualisation each offer unique methods of achieving relaxation and reducing stress. Experiment with different techniques to find what works best for you, and make a conscious effort to prioritise relaxation in your daily life. By dedicating time to relax and unwind, you can enhance your happiness and create a positive, calm state of being.

Exercise programme ideas

This chapter is slightly different as it is less about reading, more about action! I have created a series of gym-based and home-based programmes that are designed to inspire and be helpful.

Programme plan explanation

Each programme is separated into different columns – most are obvious as to what they are i.e. the exercise name. But the 'tempo' column requires a bit of explanation. The number indicates the number of seconds you have to perform the exercise. For example, "1-0-1-0" for a biceps curl means 1-second curl up, 1-second curl down. But 1-1-1-1 means 1-second curl up, 1-second hold up, 1-second curl down, 1-second stay down. The rest time stated is just a guide as well – you can take longer or go straight into the next set if you want to.

All of the programmes are generic. As your personal trainer, I would tailor your programme to your personal needs – please book an appointment if you feel that would be beneficial. I offer face-to-face or online consultations. My contact details are at the end of this book. However, I have separated the programmes into basic, intermediate and advanced. Pick where you think your fitness levels lie and give it a go. If your fitness levels exceed the advanced programmes, you can always add more weight or change the tempo to make it even harder.

These programmes are just examples of what can be added to your weekly fitness regime. There are many more sessions that are demonstrated 'on demand' in the Live Happy app.

Scan the QR code or go to https://vimeo.com/showcase/9744508 to see the exercises demonstrated!

Gym-based programmes

Session Plan 1 (Gym based) – Basic

SESSION	Exercise	Reps	Sets	Tempo	Rest	Suggested Weight	Notes
STRETCHING	Full body stretch out	2-3 mins	1	n/a	n/a	n/a	Start with shoulders and work way down to ankles
LOWER							
Set 1	Squats	10	2	1-0-1-0	30 seconds	Kettlebell, your choice of weight	Legs more than hip width apart, bend knees to squat down. Squat to bench if easier
	Mountain climbers	20	2	1-0-1-0	30 seconds	n/a	Make a plank shape, drive alternating knees towards chest and back again. On floor or elevate on bench if easier

Glute bridges	10	2	2-0-2-0	30 seconds	Kettlebell, dumbbell or light bar, your choice of weight	Lie on floor, bend knees, elevate hips up and down. Place weight on hips and hold gently
Set 2						
Lateral leg raises	10 each side	2	1-0-1-0	30 seconds	Resistance band	Wrap band around ankles. Whilst standing, bring straight leg out to the side and back again. Alternate leg
Machine leg curls	10	2	1-0-1-0	30 seconds	Low weight	Follow instructions on machine. Start with a very low weight and build
Machine leg extensions	10	2	1-0-1-0	30 seconds	Low weight	Follow instructions on machine. Start with a very low weight and build

SESSION	Exercise	Reps	Sets	Tempo	Rest	Suggested Weight	Notes
UPPER							
Set 1	Biceps curls	8-10	2	1-0-1-0	30 seconds	Dumbbells, your choice of weight	Hold dumbbells in hands, standing up. Bend arms and lift weights up towards shoulders then down
	Triceps extensions	8 each side	2	1-0-1-0	30 seconds	Dumbbell, your choice of weight	Hold onto dumbbell with one hand, hinge body at hips and place other hand down on bench. Bend weighted arm at elbow and push backwards whilst straightening. Alternate arms

	Weighted sit-ups	8-10	2	1-0-1-0	30 seconds	Dumbbell, your choice of weight	Sit on floor. Hold onto weight. Curl back onto floor and up again. Push weight forward to help lift up
Set 2	Overhead press	8-10	2	1-0-1-0	30 seconds	Low dumbbell weights or light bar	Start with weights in hands and to shoulders. Press weights up over head and back down again
	Chest press	8-10	2	1-0-1-0	30 seconds	Low dumbbell weights or light bar	Lie on bench or floor with dumbbells in hands. Create fork shape with arms then push arms together making them straight, over chest
	Russian twists	8-10	2	1-0-1-0	30 seconds	No weight or low weight	Sit on floor, legs bent and together. Lean slightly back and twist from side to side

Session Plan 2 (Gym based) – Basic

SESSION	Exercise	Reps	Sets	Tempo	Rest	Suggested Weight	Notes
STRETCHING	Full body stretch out	2–3 mins	1	n/a	n/a	n/a	Start with shoulders and work way down to ankles
CARDIO							
Set 1	Treadmill	10 minutes	2	n/a	60 seconds	n/a	Fast paced walk with slight elevation
	Star jumps	30 seconds	5	1-0-1-0	30 seconds	n/a	Standing. Arms and legs moving out and back at pace. Jump or walk
	Arm push outs	30 seconds	5	1-0-1-0	30 seconds	Very low dumbbell weights	Stand with straight arms out to side. Push arms in and out towards and away from body at pace. Weights optional

MOVE

Set 2	Bike	10 minutes	2	n/a	60 seconds	n/a	Lower level resistance
	Upright rows	30 seconds	5	1-0-1-0	30 seconds	Low weight kettlebell	Hold kettlebell with both hands, bend at elbows and draw kettlebell up towards chin, keeping elbows high and wide
	Scissor jumps	30 seconds	5	1-0-1-0	30 seconds	n/a	Jump legs back and forth at pace, creating a scissor pattern with legs
CORE							
Set 1	Bird-dog	10 each side	2	2-0-2-0	30 seconds	n/a	Start on all fours. Lift one leg straight up and out at a 90 degree angle. At the same time, lift opposite arm up and out at a 90 degree angle. Alternate arm and leg

SESSION	Exercise	Reps	Sets	Tempo	Rest	Suggested Weight	Notes
	Weighted front raises	10	2	2-0-2-0	30 seconds	Low weight kettlebell or weight plate	Start standing with weight in hands and long arms. Lift arms to 90 degree angle and back down
	Plank	20 seconds	2	n/a	30 seconds	n/a	Lie down, tummy on floor. Lift onto hands or forearms – create straight plank shape with body. Hold
Set 2	Ankles	10	2	1-0-1-0	30 seconds	n/a	Lie with back on floor. Lift head, reach round for alternating ankle at pace

Knees	10	2	1-0-1-0	30 seconds	n/a	Lie with back on floor. Lift head, reach arms up to knees and crunch, at pace
Toes	10	2	1-0-1-0	30 seconds	n/a	Lie with back on floor. Lift straight legs up to 90 degrees then reach up to toes and crunch, at pace

Session Plan 1 (Gym based) – Intermediate

SESSION	Exercise	Reps	Sets	Tempo	Rest	Suggested Weight	Notes
WARM UP	Stretching exercises	5 mins	1	n/a	n/a	n/a	Full body
	Bike or Treadmill	5 mins	1	low	n/a	Max mid level	Warm up effort only
LOWER							
Set 1	Weighted squat	10-12	2	2-0-2-0	30 seconds	Bar or kettlebell, your choice of weight	Sit down to chair if easier
	Jefferson curls	5-6	2	3-0-3-0	30 seconds	Dumbbells, your choice of weight	Roll down to floor and up slowly, keeping weights to front of legs
	Glute thrusters	10	2	1-0-2-0	30 seconds	Bar or kettlebell, your choice of weight	Bench or floor. Put weights on hips. If uncomfortable, add towel/pad

Set 2						
3/4 squats	10	2	2-0-2-0	30 seconds	Kettlebell, your choice of weight	Elevate heels on weightplate. Squat low but don't come all the way up to standing
Cable side kicks	10 each side	2	1-0-1-0	30 seconds	Cable machine, ankle attachment, your choice of weight	From standing, straight leg out to one side. Try to keep upright posture
Weighted donkey kicks	10 each side	2	2-0-2-0	30 seconds	Dumbbell, your choice of weight	Start on all fours. Tuck dumbbell in back of knee, keep knee bent, lift to 90 degrees. To progress, add resistance band around legs

SESSION	Exercise	Reps	Sets	Tempo	Rest	Suggested Weight	Notes
UPPER							
Set 3	Overhead press	8-10	2	2-0-2-0	30 seconds	Bar or dumbbells, your choice of weight	Standing, keep glutes and core activated to avoid back activating
	Triceps dips	12-15	2	1-0-1-0	30 seconds	n/a	Use bench or on floor
	21's biceps curls	7,7,7	2	1-0-1-0	30 seconds	Dumbbells, your choice of weight	Curl half way up, then top half, then all the way up and down
Set 4	Bent over rows	8-10 each side	2	2-0-2-0	30 seconds	Kettlebell, your choice of weight	Hand and knee on bench, hinge over, bend arm and pull kettlebell up towards hip

| Chest press | 10-12 | 2 | 2-0-2-0 | 30 seconds | Dumbbells, your choice of weight | Back on floor, elbows touch floor, semi-circle up and down |
| Arnie press | 6-8 | 2 | 2-0-2-0 | 30 seconds | Dumbbells, your choice of weight | Press overhead in semi-circle |

Session Plan 2 (Gym based) – Intermediate

SESSION	Exercise	Reps	Sets	Tempo	Rest	Suggested Weight	Notes
WARM UP	Stretching exercises	5 mins	1	n/a	n/a	n/a	Full body
	Bike or Treadmill	5 mins	1	low	n/a	Max mid level	Warm up effort only
Antagonists: Chest/Back							
Set 1	Bench elevated rear delt flyes	10-12	2	2-0-2-0	30 seconds	Dumbbells, your choice of weight	Face forward on bench, fly arms out to sides
	Bench elevated lat rows	10-12	2	2-0-2-0	30 seconds	Dumbbells, your choice of weight	Face forward on bench. Keep shoulders pinned back, bring weights back towards your hips

	Reps	Sets	Tempo	Rest	Equipment	Notes
Bench dumbbell chest press	10-12	2	2-0-2-0	30 seconds	Dumbbells, your choice of weight	Arms straight up, then create fork shape with arms. Don't go past 90 degrees with arms
Bench dumbbell chest flyes	10-12	2	2-0-2-0	30 seconds	Dumbbells, your choice of weight	Arms straight up then keep fairly straight, hands parallel. Don't go past 90 degrees with arms
Antagonists: Quads/ Hamstrings						
Set 2						
Leg press	10	2	2-0-2-0	30 seconds	Leg press machine, your choice of weight	Don't lock legs out. Straight at top

SESSION	Exercise	Reps	Sets	Tempo	Rest	Suggested Weight	Notes
	Backwards lunges with bar	8 each side	2	2-0-2-0	30 seconds	Bar, your choice of weight	Use core to keep balance, bar on shoulders
	Romanian deadlifts (RDLs)	10	2	2-0-2-0	30 seconds	Dumbbells or bar, your choice of weight	To progress, perform on one leg at a time
	Bulgarian split squats	8 each side	2	2-0-2-0	30 seconds	Dumbbells or bar, your choice of weight	Elevate foot using bench, keep back straight
Antagonists: Biceps/Triceps							
Set 3	Single arm biceps curls	12 each side	2	1-0-1-0	30 seconds	Dumbbell, your choice of weight	Standing or seated

Cable triceps pull downs	12-15	2	1-0-1-0	30 seconds	Cable machine, rope attachment, your choice of weight	Slight hinge at hips, keep elbows in
Bar curls	12	2	1-0-1-0	30 seconds	Cable machine bar attachment or barbell, your choice of weight	Keep glutes and core activated to stop back activating
Mini paralette narrow press ups	15-20	2	1-0-1-0	30 seconds	Mini paralette bars	Keep elbows right next to ribs. If no paralettes, perform on floor

SESSION	Exercise	Reps	Sets	Tempo	Rest	Suggested Weight	Notes
CORE							
Set 4	Bicycle crunches	20	2	2-0-2-0	30 seconds	n/a	Keep slow pace
	Leg lifts	10	2	3-0-3-0	30 seconds	n/a	On bench or floor. Keep slow pace and legs straight if possible
	Oblique crunches (left and right)	15 each side	2	1-0-1-0	30 seconds	n/a	Keep legs together, twist and make sure working oblique muscles
	Sit-ups	10	2	1-0-1-0	30 seconds	n/a	To progress, lift feet off floor
	Plank hold	40 seconds	2	n/a	30 seconds	n/a	Keep core activated to avoid back bowing

Session Plan 1 (Gym based) – Advanced

SESSION	Exercise	Reps	Sets	Tempo	Rest	Suggested Weight	Notes
WARMUP	Stretching exercises	5 mins	1	n/a	n/a	n/a	Full body
	Bike/ treadmill	5 mins	1	low	n/a	Max mid level	Warm up effort only, walking pace
Chest/Back							
	Lat pull downs	8-10	3	2-0-2-0	60 seconds	Cable machine, your choice of weight	Little arch in back and engage core
	Chin ups	8-10	3	1-0-1-0	60 seconds	Pull up bar, your choice of weight	To regress, use band to assist
	Bench chest press	8-10	3	2-0-2-0	60 seconds	Squat rack, your choice of weight	Little arch in back and engage core

SESSION	Exercise	Reps	Sets	Tempo	Rest	Suggested Weight	Notes
Quads/Hammies							
	RDLs	8-10	3	2-0-2-0	60 seconds	Bar or dumbbells, your choice of weight	Soft legs, back straight. Bar or dumbbells
	Deadlifts	6-8	3	2-0-2-0	60 seconds	Bar, your choice of weight	Pay attention to form – no pain in back, back straight
	Machine curls and extensions	8-10 each side	3	2-0-2-0	60 seconds	Machine, your choice of weight	Do quads and hamstrings
	Leg press	6-8	3	2-0-2-0	60 seconds	Machine, your choice of weight	Don't lock legs straight at top

Biceps/Triceps						
Isolated single arm curls	6–8 each side	3	2-0-2-0	60 seconds	Dumbbell, your choice of weight	Rest elbow on leg, bring weight up to chest
Half curl and hold	6–8	3	2-5-2-0	60 seconds	Dumbbells, your choice of weight	Keep posture correct as back can bow
Triceps pull downs	8–10	3	2-0-2-0	60 seconds	Cable rope attachment, your choice of weight	To progress, pull down and hold at bottom for a few seconds
CORE						
Bicycle crunches	20	2	3-0-3-0	20 seconds	n/a	Keep pace slow
Elevated bench leg lifts	10	2	2-0-2-0	20 seconds	n/a	Elevate bench, leg lift and add glute lift as well if possible

SESSION	Exercise	Reps	Sets	Tempo	Rest	Suggested Weight	Notes
	Cable oblique twists	10 each side	2	3-0-1-0	20 seconds	Cable machine, your choice of weight	Keep hips facing forward, twist at trunk
	Hanging pike	10	2	2-0-2-0	20 seconds	n/a	Hang from pull up bar, straight legs to lift towards chest

Session Plan 2 (Gym based) – Advanced

SESSION	Exercise	Reps	Sets	Tempo	Rest	Suggested Weight	Notes
WARM UP	Stretching exercises	5 mins	1	n/a	n/a	n/a	Full body
	Bike/ treadmill	5 mins	1	low	n/a	Max mid level	Warm up effort only, walking pace
PUSH							
Chest	Dumbbell chest press	10	3	2-0-2-0	30 seconds	Dumbbells, your choice of weight	Keep arms at 90 degree angle, use bench
	Dumbbell chest flyes	10	3	2-0-2-0	30 seconds	Dumbbells, your choice of weight	Keep arms wide, hands parallel
	Cable chest flyes	10	3	2-0-2-0	30 seconds	Cable machine, your choice of weight	Cable mid height, keep arms wide

SESSION	Exercise	Reps	Sets	Tempo	Rest	Suggested Weight	Notes
Shoulders	Arnie press	6-8	3	1-0-1-0	30 seconds	Dumbbells, your choice of weight	Standing or seated. Twist arms up to form semi-circle
	Overhead press	8-10	3	1-0-1-0	30 seconds	Dumbbells or bar, your choice of weight	Standing or seated
	Cable shoulder press	8-10	3	1-0-1-0	30 seconds	Cable machine, handle attachments, your choice of weight	Standing or seated
Triceps	Bench dips	12-15	3	1-0-1-0	30 seconds	n/a	Legs straight if possible

Cable triceps extensions	10 per side	3	1-0-1-0	30 seconds	Cable machine, rope attachment. your choice of weight	Slight hip hinge and keep back straight
PULL						
Back/Traps						
Pull ups	5	3	2-0-2-0	30 seconds	Pull up bar	To regress, add a resistiance band to aid
Cable rows	10	3	2-0-2-0	30 seconds	Cable machine, your choice of weight	Sit on bench, pull handle attachments down towards hips, squeeze shoulders
Bar rows	10	3	2-0-2-0	30 seconds	Bar, your choice of weight	Start standing, hinge at hip ideally at 90 degrees, pull bar up towards ribs

SESSION	Exercise	Reps	Sets	Tempo	Rest	Suggested Weight	Notes
	Rear delt flyes	10	3	2-0-2-0	30 seconds	Dumbbells, your choice of weight	Hinge at hips to 90 degrees if possible, slowly fly arms out sideways
	Cable shrugs	10	3	1-0-1-0	30 seconds	Cable machine, handle attachments, your choice of weight	Can use dumbbells or kettlebells as alternative weights
Biceps	Seated dumbbell curls	10	3	2-0-2-0	30 seconds	Dumbbells, your choice of weight	Weights to the outside of legs, keep core activated
	Bar curls	8-10	3	2-0-2-0	30 seconds	Bar, your choice of weight	Standing. Keep back straight and core/glutes activated

	Exercise	Reps	Sets	Tempo	Rest	Equipment	Notes
	Zottman curls	10	3	2-0-2-0	30 seconds	Dumbbells, your choice of weight	Curl with twist as lifting
LEGS/CORE							
Quads	Bulgarian split squats	10 per side	3	1-0-1-0	30 seconds	Dumbbells or kettlebells, your choice of weight	Foot flat or toes curled, use bench
	Walking lunges	Length of gym	3	1-0-1-0	30 seconds	Dumbbells or kettlebells, your choice of weight	Hold weights down, shoulders relaxed, walking length of gym and back
	Heel elevated weighted squats	10	3	1-0-1-0	30 seconds	Dumbbell or kettlebell, your choice of weight	Optional to elevate heels. Can elevate toes instead

SESSION	Exercise	Reps	Sets	Tempo	Rest	Suggested Weight	Notes
Hamstrings	Good mornings	6-8	3	3-1-3-0	30 seconds	Bar, your choice of weight	Back straight, hinge over as far as you can
	Leg curls	8-10	3	2-0-2-0	30 seconds	Machine or cable (ankle attachment), your choice of weight	To progress, try single leg on machine
	Kettlebell swings	12-15	3	1-0-1-0	30 seconds	Kettlebell, your choice of weight	Hip hinge, glute squeeze, keep back straight
Glutes	Cable donkey kicks	10 each side	3	1-0-1-0	30 seconds	Cable machine, ankle attachment, your choice of weight	Slight hip hinge, make sure weight is backwards and on standing leg

Exercise	Reps	Sets	Tempo	Rest	Equipment	Notes
Single leg RDLs	8 each side	3	2-0-2-0	30 seconds	Dumbbell or landmine bar, your choice of weight	Slight hip hinge, make sure weight is backwards and on standing leg
Glute bridges	12-15	3	2-0-2-0	30 seconds	Bar, your choice of weight	Curl spine up and down, squeeze glutes
CORE						
Bench v-sits	30	3	1-0-1-0	30 seconds	n/a	Sit on bench, hold on, lift legs, bring legs straight and bent
Boat pose	30 seconds	3	1-0-1-0	30 seconds	n/a	Sit on floor, elevate straight legs and arms, then hold
Side plank dips	15 each side	3	1-0-1-0	30 seconds	n/a	Make sure hips stacked and not too much pressure on shoulder

SESSION	Exercise	Reps	Sets	Tempo	Rest	Suggested Weight	Notes
CARDIO – HIIT	Burpees	40 seconds	5	1-0-1-0	20 seconds	n/a	To progress, add jump and press up
	Press ups	40 seconds	5	1-0-1-0	20 seconds	n/a	To progress, lift alternate foot off floor
	Front punches	40 seconds	5	1-0-1-0	20 seconds	n/a	To progress, hold onto dumbbell weights
	Air squats	40 seconds	5	1-0-1-0	20 seconds	n/a	To progress, hold onto weight

Home-based programmes
Session Plan 1 (no equipment) – Basic

SESSION	Exercise	Reps	Sets	Tempo	Rest	Notes
WARM UP	Calf raises	10	2	1-0-1-0	20 seconds	Hold on to the back of a chair and lift onto toes
	Fast marches	20 seconds	2	1-0-1-0	20 seconds	Move arms as well as legs
	Child's pose push throughs	8	2	2-0-2-0	20 seconds	Start in child's pose, move head and hips forward into a cobra position, then reverse back to child's pose
	Star steps	10	2	1-0-1-0	20 seconds	Similar to star jumps but step feet out as opposed to jumping
BODY WEIGHT	Box press ups	10	3	1-0-1-0	40-60 seconds	Start on all fours, bend arms and bring face towards the floor, then straighten arms back up

SESSION	Exercise	Reps	Sets	Tempo	Rest	Notes
	Triceps dips on a chair	10	3	1-0-1-0	40-60 seconds	Sit on chair, place hands on chair with elbows facing backwards, slip bottom off chair and bend at elbows then push back up
	Side lunges	5 each side	3	2-0-2-0	40-60 seconds	Step far out to one side and bend knee to lunge. Repeat on the other side
	Donkey kicks	10 each side	3	2-0-2-0	40-60 seconds	Start on all fours, left bent leg up behind to a 90 degree angle. Alternate legs
	Squats with a pulse	10	3	1-0-1-0	40-60 seconds	Squat to chair and add a little pulse at the bottom of squat

CARDIO					
High knees	30 seconds	3	1-0-1-0	20 seconds	Try to keep as fast as possible but slow to a walk if struggling
Butt kicks	30 seconds	3	1-0-1-0	20 seconds	Try to keep as fast as possible but slow to a walk if struggling
CORE					
Crunches	10	3	1-0-1-0	30 seconds	Lie with back on floor. Hands behind head and lift shoulders and head off the floor
Heel touches	10 each side	3	1-0-1-0	30 seconds	Lie with back on floor. Lift head and shoulders off the floor, then reach round to each side of ankles

Session Plan 2 (no equipment) - Basic

SESSION	Exercise	Reps	Sets	Tempo	Rest	Notes
WARM UP	Lateral raised circles	10 each way	2	1-0-1-0	20 seconds	Arms straight out to sides and rotate arms clockwise and anti-clockwise
	Front punches	20	2	1-0-1-0	20 seconds	Make fists and punch arms forwards, alternately
	Downward dog raise on to toes	10	2	2-0-2-0	20 seconds	Start on all fours and raise bottom into a downward dog position, then raise onto toes and back down again
	Roll up roll downs	5	2	1-0-1-0	20 seconds	Gently roll down, hinging at hips and try to touch the floor with hands. Roll back up again to starting position

UPPER					
Kitchen work surface press ups	10	3	2-0-2-0	40-60 seconds	Place hands on work surface to create plank shape. Bend elbows moving face towards work surface. Keep body straight
Coffee table shoulder taps	20	3	2-0-2-0	40-60 seconds	Place hands on coffee table to create plank shape. Alternately lift one hand off surface and tap opposite shoulder
Kitchen work surface dips	30	3	4-0-4-0	40-60 seconds	Face away from cupboards and surface with back touching. Place hands on surface, elbows facing backwards. Bend at elbows and dip down.

SESSION	Exercise	Reps	Sets	Tempo	Rest	Notes
LOWER	Kitchen work surface squats	10	3	2-0-2-0	40-60 seconds	Place hands on work surface. Squat down using surface to assist balance
	Kitchen work surface lateral leg raises	10 each side	3	1-0-1-0	40-60 seconds	Use work surface to balance. Lift straight leg out and back
	Forward lunges	10	3	1-0-1-0	40-60 seconds	Step forwards, bend at knee. Travel forwards around room
CORE	Bent leg lowers	10	2	3-0-3-0	30 seconds	Lie on back and place hands under bottom, then lower bent legs up and down
	Pencil to ball crunches	5	2	1-0-1-0	30 seconds	Lie on back and bring knees to chest, then stretch arms and legs out to create long pencil shape

Session Plan 1 (no equipment) – Intermediate

SESSION	Exercise	Reps	Sets	Tempo	Rest	Notes
WARM UP	Squats to calf raises	15	1	1-0-1-0	20 seconds	Squat down then lift heels off floor
	Lat raises to front raises	15	1	1-0-1-0	20 seconds	Lift straight arms forward then to sides
	Inch worms	5	1	3-0-3-0	20 seconds	Also called plank walk outs. Start standing, walk out to plank then walk back up
	Hamstring leg sweeps	10 each side	1	2-0-2-0	20 seconds	Also called 'feed the chickens'. From standing, hinge forward and sweep hands along floor height, then back up to stand again

SESSION	Exercise	Reps	Sets	Tempo	Rest	Notes
UPPER	Press up variation 1	5 each leg	3	2-0-2-0	60 seconds	One foot in air when performing press ups
	Plank twists	10 each arm	3	2-0-2-0	60 seconds	Plank with twist to alternating hip touching floor
	Press up variation 2	10	3	2-0-2-0	60 seconds	Downward dog to press up
LOWER	Jump squats with floor touch	10	3	2-0-2-0	60 seconds	Squat, reach hand down and touch floor, jump up. To regress, don't jump
	Side lunges	10 each side	3	1-0-1-0	60 seconds	Step to side. Alternate legs, try at pace
	Jumping split squats	10	3	1-0-1-0	60 seconds	Alternate legs, one leg forwards, one backwards, try at pace. To regress, don't jump

CORE					
Leg levers	8	3	3-0-3-0	30 seconds	Lie on back, hands under glutes. Keep legs straight if possible
Side crunches	10 each side	3	1-0-1-0	30 seconds	Lie on back, twist legs to one side. Hands behind head and crunch
Spiderman plank holds	20 seconds each side	3	N/A	30 seconds	Plank position, draw knee in towards arms, alternating legs

Session Plan 2 (no equipment) – Intermediate

SESSION	Exercise	Reps	Sets	Tempo	Rest	Notes
High Intensity	High knees	40 seconds	3	1-0-1-0	20 seconds	To regress, change to a fast march
	Jump squats	40 seconds	3	1-0-1-0	20 seconds	To regress, remove jump
	Butt kicks	40 seconds	3	1-0-1-0	20 seconds	To regress, remove jump
	Front punches	40 seconds	3	1-0-1-0	20 seconds	To progress, add small weights
	Mountain climbers	40 seconds	3	1-0-1-0	20 seconds	To regress, remove jumps or slow down
	Alternating plank	40 seconds	3	1-0-1-0	20 seconds	To regress, perform on knees instead of toes
LOWER – holds	Chair pose	40 seconds	3	n/a	60 seconds	To progress, perform exercise on one leg

UPPER – holds					
Wall sit	60 seconds	3	n/a	60 seconds	To progress, add weight
Plank hold	60 seconds	3	n/a	30 seconds	To regress, plank hold on knees
Inverted bridge hold	40 seconds	3	n/a	30 seconds	Use floor or chair. To progress, straighten legs
CORE					
Bicycle crunches	20	3	2-0-2-0	30 seconds	Keep slower pace, stretch leg out fully and elbow to opposite knee
Russian twists	20	3	2-0-2-0	30 seconds	To progress, hover feet off floor
Scissors	10	3	3-0-3-0	30 seconds	Place hands under glutes to steady back, keep alternating legs at slow pace

SESSION	Exercise	Reps	Sets	Tempo	Rest	Notes
	Flutter kicks	30 seconds	3	1-0-1-0	30 seconds	Keep alternating straight legs at pace. To regress, bring straight legs further up towards 90 degree angle

Session Plan 1 (no equipment) – Advanced

SESSION	Exercise	Reps	Sets	Tempo	Rest	Notes
WARM UP	Front punches	20	2	1-0-1-0	20 seconds	Add small dumbbell weights to intensify if you have them
	Squat pulses	20	2	1-0-1-0	20 seconds	1 second pulse at bottom of squat
	Bent leg windscreen wipers	5 each side	2	3-0-3-0	20 seconds	Straighten legs to intensify
BODY WEIGHT	Triceps dips	10	3	2-0-2-0	30 seconds	Legs straight, hold at bottom of move for one second
	Burpees	20	3	2-0-2-0	30 seconds	To progress, add in more explosive star jump and press up
	Chest to ground press ups	30	3	2-0-2-0	30 seconds	To progress, add hand claps in between press ups

SESSION	Exercise	Reps	Sets	Tempo	Rest	Notes
	Lunge jumps	40	3	2-0-2-0	30 seconds	20 each leg
	Mountain climbers	50	3	1-0-1-0	30 seconds	On floor or bench
	Wall sit	60 seconds	3	N/A	30 seconds	To progress, add weight if available
	Crow pose hold	20 seconds	3	N/A	30 seconds	Balancing on hands
	Handstand against wall hold	20 seconds	3	N/A	30 seconds	To regress, try headstand
INTERVAL CARDIO	Sprint-jog	10 seconds	10	1-0-1-0	20 seconds	Outside – sprint for 10 seconds then jog for 20 seconds
CORE	X-man crunch	10	3	1-0-1-0	30 seconds	Try to keep legs and arms elevated
	Reverse crunches	20	3	1-0-1-0	30 seconds	Try to keep legs and arms elevated

Elevated feet Russian twists	20 (each side)	3	1-0-1-0	30 seconds	To progress, add weight if available
Seated abs circles	10 each way	3	2-0-2-0	30 seconds	Clockwise and anti-clockwise
Sit-up twists	20	3	1-0-1-0	30 seconds	Alternating sides

Session Plan 2 (no equipment) – Advanced

SESSION	Exercise	Reps	Sets	Tempo	Rest	Notes
WARM UP	Jump squats	25	2	1-0-1-0	20 seconds	To regress, lose jump
	Hand release press ups	20	2	1-0-1-0	20 seconds	Chest to ground press up then lift hands before reversing
	Sumo heel lifts	15	2	1-0-1-0	20 seconds	Alternate each heel lift or together
	Explosive star jumps	10	2	1-0-1-0	20 seconds	To regress, switch to usual star jumps
UPPER	Archer press ups	10 each side	4	2-0-2-0	30 seconds	To regress, switch to wide press ups
	Plank alternating toe touches	10 each side	4	1-0-1-0	30 seconds	Plank to downward dog to toe touch, then reverse
	Bear walks	Room length	4	1-0-1-0	30 seconds	Walk length of room forwards then backwards

LOWER	Frog squats	10	4	1-0-1-0	30 seconds	To progress, add jump at top
	Pistol squats	10 each side	4	2-0-2-0	30 seconds	To regress, squat to bench
	Pulsing jumping lunges	10	4	1-0-1-0	30 seconds	To regress, lose pulse
CORE	Leg levers	15	3	3-0-3-0	30 seconds	Keep slow pace up and down
	V-sit hold	30 second hold	3	1-0-1-0	30 seconds	To regress, bend legs
	Side plank leg lift	15 each side	3	N/A	30 seconds	To regress, just hold side plank

EAT

"You are what you eat! To stay healthy we need more than 40 different nutrients. No single food can provide them all." (The Happiness Project)

I thought it best not to bombard you with too much scientific detail as it can get complex when it comes to the fuel we humans consume, but this section of the book aims to answer some common questions and provide you with information about the basics of nutrition. If you are trying to eat better and feel better but get easily overwhelmed by the wave of information on the internet, or simply don't know where to start, then this will help. I finish this section with some tried-and-tested recipe ideas for healthy eating, to make it easier for you to put the theory into practice.

What is a balanced diet?

We're all told to eat a balanced diet, or at least to aim for one, but what is a balanced diet?

This chapter provides a brief overview of all the components of a balanced diet, dispels a few myths, and gives you clarity on the basics of what should be on your plate at dinner time.

A balanced diet is simply about eating the correct proportions of the different food groups that your body needs to function. It doesn't mean that you are 'on a diet' and reducing your calorie intake. An overconsumption of one group at the expense of another can upset your body's delicate balance. Food gives us nutrients that cells and systems in our bodies need, as well as non-nutrients essential for health, such as fibre and water.

Macro-nutrients

Let's start with the main larger categories: carbohydrates, protein and fats. These are macronutrients. If you've ever heard the term 'macros', this is what it refers to. We need carbohydrates, protein and fats in large quantities which are used for structure and function, and to fuel our bodies.

Carbohydrates

Putting it simply, carbohydrates give us energy. They also provide nutrients like calcium, iron, and B vitamins, as well as fibre, which is essential for digestive health. Carbs can be broken down into three categories: complex carbs (rice, bread, pasta, potatoes, and vegetables), simple carbs (fruits, sugar, honey, and fruit juice), and fibre (fruit and vegetables).

Protein

This macro is important for growth and repair and is often discussed in the gym with regard to helping your muscles repair after a workout. Protein is made up of amino acids which are the building blocks of your body. They are used to rebuild the body's structures: muscle, tendons, ligaments, and bone. Protein is also the main component of your skin, organs, and most bodily fluids. We constantly break down and use protein in every cell of our body so it's important to have a regular supply. Great sources of natural protein include eggs, chicken, and soy products.

Fats

Fats are often vilified, as too much can raise cholesterol levels, but they are a vital component of a healthy diet and have several important functions. Fats provide you with energy and are also used for insulation and protection of your organs. They're essential for the transportation and use of vitamins, they help with hormone and enzyme production, and they support both your immune system and your central nervous system. There are a number of different types of fats: saturated (such as butter), unsaturated (such as avocado), and trans fats (such as doughnuts). It's important to know which is which, to eat the right amounts of both saturated and unsaturated fats, and to try to avoid trans fats.

Micronutrients

These are vitamins and minerals. We need these in smaller quantities than macros to support and manage some of the vital processes in the body. They don't provide energy but our bodies need them to survive as we can't produce them on our own. Vitamins and minerals allow chemical reactions to happen within your body, allowing your immune, hormonal, and nervous systems to function properly. We also need them to be able to use the energy contained within macronutrients, and we need specific minerals and vitamins for specific functions. A varied diet is an easy way to eat a wide range.

Water

Although it's not a nutrient, it's still essential for health and performance. Your body can survive for several weeks without food, but can only manage for about three days without water. Water must be present to support life because it helps cells function and sustains reactions within the body. It also helps to maintain and form blood plasma, which is 90% of the liquid portion of blood. That's why, when you get dehydrated, your blood volume falls, meaning that it can carry less oxygen around your body, and that's why you feel tired! Making sure you drink the recommended guidelines for water not only helps everything inside your body work properly, but it can also make you feel better!

Summary

Consuming varied sources of carbohydrates, proteins, fats, vitamins, minerals, and enough water to provide your body with all the things it needs to keep you functioning and feeling healthy, is a balanced diet. The UK/NHS Live Well Eatwell Guide provides easy-to-follow information on the quantities we should be aiming to eat from each food group to achieve a balanced diet. The next few chapters delve into more detail about each of the macro and micronutrients.

The basics

This chapter delves a little deeper into the different food groups, to give a bit more clarity to what you are fuelling your body with.

Carbohydrates

Carbs often get a bad rep! Put simply, carbohydrates are your body's main source of energy, but they also keep your digestive system healthy. They come in two main types: simple carbohydrates and complex carbohydrates.

At a very simple level, when you eat carbohydrates, they get broken down to create glucose. Glucose enters your bloodstream, fuels your brain and your muscles, and helps your cells to function. We need to eat them regularly to keep our energy levels consistent and allow our bodies to function properly. The difference between simple and complex carbs is how long they take to get broken down into glucose.

Simple carbs

All carbohydrates are like a wall made up of small bricks (or units of sugars, called saccharides). The bigger the wall, the harder it is to break it down into individual bricks. Simple carbs only have a few bricks in the wall; they can be single or double sugar units, which easily get broken down into glucose and into your bloodstream quickly to provide your body with easily accessible energy.

Natural sources include fruit, milk, and honey. Natural simple carbs come in a more nutritious package for your body as they also have vitamins, minerals, water, and fibre (all good things your body likes). Processed sources of simple carbs include biscuits, cakes, confectionery, and soft drinks. These are less nutritious and often contain high levels of sugar, fat, and artificial sweeteners.

Complex carbs

Complex carbs are bigger walls, with more bricks in them. They are made up of lots of sugar units bound together to create larger structures. This means they take longer to be broken down, providing a slower release of glucose and a more sustained source of energy. To avoid constant highs and lows of your blood sugar levels, it's a good idea to include complex carbs in your diet.

Natural unrefined sources of complex carbs include wholemeal and wholegrains, vegetables, and pulses such as kidney beans, chickpeas, and soybeans. Again, along with the energy, they also contain vitamins, minerals, antioxidants, and fibre. These sorts of unrefined complex carbs are the preferred choice: they are more like natural carbs and are overall more nutritious for the functioning of the body.

Refined complex carbs include white bread, pasta, cakes, biscuits, and pastries. As these foodstuffs have been processed, they often contain high levels of sugar and low-quality fats, and are less nutritious as fibre, vitamins, and minerals have been extracted.

The problems with carbohydrates start when you eat too many of them. Once your body's energy requirements have been fulfilled and glucose has been stored away in your muscles and liver, the rest can float around your body looking for somewhere to settle down. The excess gets converted into fat and is deposited in your adipose tissues for long-term energy storage, resulting in weight gain.

Fibre

Fibre is the other important thing we get from carbohydrates. It's the indigestible plant material from complex carbs like fruits, veg, beans, and grains. It isn't used for energy as we can't break it down but it's still vital for a healthy body. It allows an easy flow of the digestive system. A combination of suitable amounts of fibre and hydration will make you more regular (at least once or twice a day) – we don't want waste products hanging around inside our bodies. Fibre makes you feel fuller for longer and can help control blood cholesterol levels. It also regulates blood sugar levels because high-fibre foods take longer to break down, so glucose is released into the blood at a slower rate.

The UK/NHS Eatwell Guide recommends that starchy carbs should make up just over a third of the food we eat (including fruit and veg that makes up roughly 50-60% of your daily intake), with the emphasis on wholegrain and high-fibre options with less added salt, sugar, and fat.

Summary

Carbohydrates serve some very important functions within the body when eaten in the correct quantities. They provide energy for your brain, cells, and muscles, and contribute fibre to help with digestion, blood sugar, and satiety. So, remember to try to choose unrefined, simple and complex carbs where possible, such as fruit, veg, grains, and wholegrain/wholemeal products like pasta, rice, and bread. Not only do these foods contain more fibre, but they also contribute nutrients to your diet like vitamins, minerals, antioxidants, and water which your body will thank you for.

Protein

Every cell in your body contains protein. About three-quarters of your muscle is protein and that's about 18-20% of your body's weight. The only other substance that's more abundant is water! Protein is made up of amino acids which, when broken down through digestion, are used to grow, repair, and rebuild structures in your body. There are 20 amino acids that your body needs, 9 of which are essential to have in your diet that your body can't make on its own, and the other 11 your body can make from the essential ones if it needs to. The main source of these amino acids is from consuming protein, which comes in two types: complete and incomplete proteins.

Complete and incomplete proteins

Complete proteins have all nine essential amino acids (AAs) your body needs. Foodstuffs include eggs, meat, poultry, dairy, and fish from animal sources, and soy foods, buckwheat, and quinoa from non-animal sources. These foods are one-stop shops for all the protein AAs you need. Incomplete proteins come from plant foods and lack one or more essential AA. These include pulses, vegetables, nuts, seeds, and beans.

If you eat animal products, you get everything you need from complete protein sources. But if you don't, then you need to eat a wide range of plant-based proteins and think about balancing your sources to get the nine essential AAs from different complementary incomplete proteins. There's no disadvantage to doing this as it doesn't matter where you get them from, as long as you're getting everything you need naturally.

What do amino acids do?

Amino acids build structures within the body, repair muscle tissue, and build skin cells. They also help with the overall function of the body, including aiding hormone, enzyme, and white blood cell production. The quality of these structures depends on the quality of the protein you eat, so try to make sure you are eating good quality protein where possible. The least processed or refined products usually provide a more complete and high-quality source of nutrients.

How much protein should I be eating?

The recommended starting point is that about 15-20% of your diet should be made up of protein and should make up a major part of every meal. Two or three protein-rich food servings meet the needs of most adults each day. The Eatwell Guide recommends at least two portions of fish every week, one of which should be oily, like salmon or mackerel. Lean meat or mince should be chosen, as well as less red and processed meat like bacon, ham, and sausages. Eggs are also a good source of protein, as well as a range of other vitamins and minerals. Pulses like beans, peas, and lentils are another great source, as well as being lower in fat and higher in fibre than meat.

The amount your body needs varies depending on your gender, due to body composition. On average, men have more muscle mass than women due to their higher levels of testosterone. Your need for protein also increases with age. In addition, it is a good idea to have more protein if you are especially active, to help your muscles repair, or if you're pregnant, to help with the baby's growth.

For anyone concerned about the amount of protein they are consuming per day, it's worth noting that your body can't use much more than 25-35g of protein in one go. So, it's best to spread out your protein sources throughout the day, rather than trying to get it all in one meal, especially if you're trying to consume more protein to help build muscle or lose weight. Research has shown that a diet which distributes 90g of protein evenly between breakfast, lunch, and dinner stimulated muscle protein synthesis (or muscle repair) to a greater degree than when the largest portion of protein was eaten at dinner. (Mamerow et al, 2014)

Summary

Protein consumption is a popular topic at the moment; you'll see it on packaging for everything from cereals to snacks to drinks, but it's worth thinking about the quality and quantity of the protein you're consuming to make sure it's in line with your body's needs. As we constantly use and lose it, we need to make sure our bodies are provided with a regular and varied supply of good quality sources of protein to keep them growing and repairing healthily.

Fats

Fats can be a tricky topic which causes a lot of confusion. Let's start by learning about what fats do in our bodies. They're essential for healthy cells, the nervous system, and the production of important hormones and enzymes. They're also extremely important for transporting, storing, and using fat-soluble vitamins A, D, E, and K. Fats also provide a source of energy during lower-intensity activity and are stored in adipose tissue for energy, as well as insulation.

Fats and oils are often referred to as lipids. Lipids which are liquid at room temperature are called oils, and those which are solid are called fats. There are two main types found in foods: saturated and unsaturated fats. The type of fat depends on the chains of fatty acids that make it up. These can be different lengths or shapes which give them different characteristics.

Saturated fat

This tends to be solid at room temperature. It's usually found in animal products like meat, poultry, dairy, and eggs. We also find it in non-animal products like coconut oil, palm oil, and cocoa butter. These fats are naturally occurring fats, so as a rule, your body knows what to do with them. They can be broken down and used by your body as a building block. We need to make sure that we eat these in moderation, as diets high in saturated fat have been linked to heart disease and other health issues.

Unsaturated fat

This tends to be liquid at room temperature. It's usually found in plants and marine animals such as olive oil, rapeseed oil, avocados, nuts, and oily fish. These fats are good for your heart, can help with cholesterol levels, and have other positive effects on the body when they replace saturated fats and are consumed in the right quantities.

Unsaturated fats can be broken down into smaller categories of monounsaturated or polyunsaturated fats. Monounsaturated fats can be found in things like lard, beef dripping, nuts, seeds, olives, avocados, and oils like rapeseed, sesame, peanut, and olive. Polyunsaturated fats include omega-3 and omega-6 fats, which are fundamental to health. They help with your metabolism and the function of your cells. They are essential fats because your body cannot make them, so we must eat them in the required amounts for good health. They have lots of health benefits for the body such as reducing blood clotting, improving cholesterol profiles, and lowering inflammation.

Sources of omega-3 are oily fish like mackerel, salmon and sardines, cod liver oil, eggs from pasture-reared hens, as well as nut and seed oils like flax, hemp, and walnut. Sources of omega-6 are oils from foodstuffs such as sunflower, corn, safflower and grapeseed, evening primrose oil, and seeds like pumpkin and sesame.

Trans fats

Trans fats or hydrogenated fats are unsaturated fatty acids which have been altered during the manufacturing process when liquid fats have been changed into solids. These are generally processed foods which we want to eat in moderation anyway (margarine products, pre-prepared meals, biscuits, cakes, pastries, and takeaways). Because they are chemically processed, our bodies struggle to know what to do with them so they often result in excessive fat storage and other health complications.

What fats should I be eating?

Around 20-30% of your energy should be coming from fats. Obviously, this should be adjusted to take your lifestyle and activity levels into account. The government recommends no more than 20-30g of saturated fat per day, and only up to 5g of trans fats per day. Unsaturated fats are encouraged and it's important to ensure that you are getting enough omega-3 and omega-6. Two portions of fish per week, one of which is oily, should help with omega-3 levels.

Summary

Ideally, we want to include a range of fat types in our diet. We should be careful about hidden or manufactured fats, especially ones which come in products that are also high in salt and sugar. We should aim for a mix of saturated, mono- and polyunsaturated fats from protein foods (meat, poultry, dairy, and fish) and added fats (butter, avocado, peanut butter, and oils). These are easily converted into energy and used throughout the body, or stored away for later, to ensure a healthy nervous system, hormone and enzyme production, and cells.

Fruit and vegetables

Fruits and vegetables should make up over a third of the food we eat each day. The UK government recommends five portions a day. Fruit and veg are important sources of fibre, as well as vitamins and minerals. They're also carbohydrates and, as such, provide us with energy.

Vegetables and fruit contain fibre, but what is fibre and why do I need it? Fibre is found in the cell walls of vegetables, fruit, pulses, and cereal grains. It can't be broken down so is indigestible but although it has no nutritional value, it is still extremely important! Firstly, it helps with the digestion process and keeps the bowels healthy. Fibre helps everything move along smoothly and regularly, meaning that waste products, which we don't want hanging around, can be removed quickly.

Fibre also makes you feel fuller for longer and helps regulate blood sugar levels, as high-fibre foods take longer to break down. This means glucose is released into the blood at a slower rate and it can also help control blood cholesterol levels.

Types of fibre

There are two types of fibre: soluble and insoluble fibre. Soluble fibre comes from the insides of fruit, veg, and pulses. It absorbs water and becomes a soft, gel-like substance. It can be partly digested and may help reduce cholesterol levels in the blood.

Insoluble fibre is tougher and doesn't dissolve. It's often left intact as it moves through the body and mainly comes from the outer shells or skins of seeds, grains, fruits, and vegetables. Keeping the skin on things like apples and sweet potatoes can be a great source of insoluble fibre which helps food and waste products to move through the body more easily. Both types are important and eating a range of fruit and veg will help you to get a decent amount of fibre in your diet, as well as all the other benefits these foods provide.

What counts as my five-a-day?

Quantities of foods vary, and you want to be aiming for a range of different types, but to give you a few examples, one portion of your five-a-day is: 80g of fresh, canned or frozen fruit or vegetables; one banana, apple or similar-sized fruit; three heaped tablespoons of vegetables; and one small bowl of salad. Some things only count once though. For example, the recommended limit per day of fruit juice, vegetable juice or a smoothie is 150ml due to high sugar content.

What source is best?

This is a question that comes up a lot – the answer is that they are all great. However you like your fruit and vegetables, whether they be fresh, frozen, tinned, dried, or juiced, they are all good. The only thing to note with juiced fruit and veg is that this can remove the fibre, which, of course, we want in our diet.

If you're struggling to eat your five portions a day, here are some easy ways to add in more:

- Add a tablespoon of dried fruit, such as raisins, to your morning cereal or porridge.

- Swap your mid-morning cereal bar for a banana or an apple with some peanut butter for a snack.

- Add a portion of salad to your lunch, or throw a portion of mixed veg into your dinner.

- Try some fruit with yoghurt for dessert.

Summary

I know it can be difficult getting enough fruit and veg into your diet each day, but it is more important than you think. As mentioned, they help to give you the vitamins and minerals your body needs, and they are packed with fibre which is vital for your digestive health and helps to control your blood sugar levels. Do your best to eat your five-a-day, as part of your balanced diet.

Vitamins and minerals

Vitamins and minerals are called micronutrients. They are not needed for energy production but are essential in small quantities to keep the body healthy. Our bodies cannot make these, so we have to get them from our food. But what do they do? Vitamins and minerals allow important chemical reactions within the body to take place. They form an important part of our cells' structures and some are essential for the enzyme system, which produces energy. Others assist our immune, hormone, and nervous systems. These are all important things.

Vitamins are formed by plants and are obtained by either eating those plants or products from animals that have eaten those plants.

Types of vitamins

Water-soluble vitamins are vitamins which are absorbed, transported, and used within water, like B vitamins and vitamin C. They can't be stored in large quantities so need to be included in your daily diet. Then we have fat-soluble vitamins A, D, E, and K. They can only be absorbed, transported, and used in the presence of fat, so not having enough fat in your diet can cause deficiencies. If you consume more than you need, the vitamins simply leave the body in urine, so again they should be included in your daily diet.

Minerals

Minerals usually occur in soil and are drawn up into plants by the roots. Our body requires minerals in varying amounts. Calcium, chloride, magnesium, potassium, and sodium are required in larger quantities, while some are only needed in small, or trace, amounts, like iodine, boron, and manganese.

Minerals have many regulatory functions, like controlling fluid balance, muscle contractions, nerve functions, hormone production, and the formation of red blood cells. Sodium and potassium are essential for the nervous system to help with muscle and nerve function. They also work together to control your body's fluid balance. Calcium is a mineral most of us know we need for strong bones and teeth, but calcium must also be present for muscle contractions to occur.

How do vitamins and minerals work?

Here are some examples of the way vitamins and minerals work together to keep you healthy:

Vitamin C is great for the immune system, which we all know is important in the cold and flu season. Vitamin C helps grow strong connective tissue, heals wounds, promotes healthy blood vessels, and is needed to produce the hormone adrenaline. It also helps with the absorption of iron, so if you eat vitamin C-rich food with iron-rich food, your body will be able to process and use more of the iron than if you had simply eaten the iron-rich food.

For example, egg yolks are a good source of iron, and tomatoes and peppers are a great source of vitamin C. So, if you were to make scrambled eggs but added in some tomatoes and peppers, you'd absorb more iron from the egg yolks because of the presence of the tomatoes and peppers than if you'd simply had the eggs on their own.

Another example is vitamin B. In order to access the energy in carbohydrates, your body needs vitamin B to be present. In order for vitamin B to be used within your body, as it is a water-soluble vitamin, you need to be well hydrated.

How do you get vitamins and minerals into your diet?

Good sources are fresh fruit and vegetables, raw nuts, legumes, pulses, unrefined wholegrains, dairy, eggs, meat, fortified products, and leafy green vegetables. Eating a wide variety of at least five portions of fruit and veg in a range of colours will provide you with a sufficiently rich array of vitamins, minerals, and other nutrients that your body needs. Try to eat vegetables that are as fresh as possible and avoid overcooking them.

If you are very active, you probably need to consume the upper limits of the quantity recommendations. You need to make sure that you have the vitamins and minerals involved in energy production and the metabolism of carbohydrates and fat, as well as those which help to encourage red blood cell production, muscle growth, and tissue repair.

Summary

As a general rule, a range of fresh fruits and veg in a rainbow of colours, as well as other nutrient-dense foods, will ensure that you're getting everything you need. If you are at all concerned, a qualified dietitian or doctor can prescribe supplements and diagnose any deficiencies.

Water and alcohol

Humans are made up of over 70% water! I am constantly asking clients how much water they are drinking in the day, and it is usually nowhere near enough. Water is not a nutrient, but it is essential for health and performance. But why?

Water enables the optimal functioning of your cells, transporting nutrients in and waste products out via the bloodstream. It also helps to maintain volume and form blood plasma, which is a large part of the liquid portion of blood. Water also lubricates joints, protects organs and tissues, and allows the maintenance of a consistent and regular body temperature. It also interacts with other elements of your diet; for example, when combined with fibre, it assists regular digestive transit, and allows water-soluble vitamins such as vitamin B, to be utilised. Making sure you drink enough water can help you to feel energised for several reasons, one being that vitamin B is involved in the conversion of carbohydrates into energy.

How much water should I be drinking?

The UK Eatwell Guide recommends 6-8 glasses of water and other liquids per day, which is roughly 1.2 to 1.5 litres. The amount you should be drinking also depends on the temperature and humidity of the environment you're in, your own body temperature, and respiration rate. If any of these are high, it's recommended to increase your water consumption. It's also generally advised to drink one extra litre of water per hour of physical activity or exercise. I usually advise my personal training clients to drink two litres per day.

Water, low-fat milk and sugar-free drinks, including tea and coffee, all count towards your daily fluid intake. Fruit juice and smoothies also count but should be limited to 150ml, as they can be a high source of sugar. If you don't like the taste of water, sugar-free squashes or slices of fruit can be an easy way to make your drinking more enjoyable.

As mentioned, tea and coffee count, but remember that if they are caffeinated, they can make you urinate more regularly, causing your hydration levels to drop.

Dehydration

Staying hydrated helps to keep your energy levels up and can generally make you feel better. Because water makes up so much of our blood, when we get dehydrated, our blood volume is lowered, meaning that there's less of it to carry oxygen and nutrients around the body that we need for energy production. That's why we can feel tired even if we've slept well and eaten enough.

Dehydration can be serious but is easily avoided. Some of the early signs are: headache, fatigue, loss of appetite, flushed skin, dry eyes, and darker coloured urine. The easiest solution is to drink little and often, continually keeping your body's water levels topped up, rather than downing half a litre in one go when you realise you are thirsty. Your body can survive for several weeks without food, but without water, it can only manage for about three days, so drink up!

Alcohol

Something I get asked as a health and well-being professional very frequently is about alcohol consumption. Should I drink at all and how much is too much? This research is from drinkaware.co.uk.

Alcohol is measured in units which is a term I'm sure you're familiar with. These units are calculated by the strength of the alcohol. One unit is the same as 10 ml or 8g of pure alcohol. Over the years, alcohol strength has increased but measures have stayed the same so you could be drinking more than you realise!

What are the alcohol consumption guidelines?

Current UK guidelines recommend no more than 14 units per week. This is the equivalent of around 6 pints of beer or 10 small glasses of wine. It's best to spread your drinking evenly over three or more days. If you have one or two heavy drinking episodes a week, you increase your risk of long-term illness and injury. Heavy or binge drinking is considered to be drinking twice the recommended daily units on one occasion, e.g. eight units in one sitting. There aren't significant risks to health if drinking within these guidelines, but if you were to drink above these recommendations regularly, it can have quite a detrimental effect on your health.

Why is it not a good idea to drink in excess?

If you drink above the guidance, you put yourself at risk of a range of short- and long-term effects on your body, lifestyle, and mental health. In the short term, these are things such as injuries and accidents, low energy, and sexual performance difficulties. It can also affect your appearance and lead to weight gain. In the long term, there can be many serious medical conditions like liver disease, hypertension, cardiovascular disease, stroke, cancers of the throat and mouth, type-2 diabetes, and brain damage. It's also associated with depression and anxiety.

What can I do to reduce my drinking?

Here are five ways that Drinkaware recommends to cut down on the amount you drink:

1. Track what you drink. You can even use the Live Happy app tracker to assist you.

2. Know the strength of what you're drinking

3. Cut down on the size of your drink. Opt for halves instead of pints, a smaller glass of wine, or a spritzer to reduce the number of units.

4. Alternate between soft drinks or water and alcoholic drinks.

5. Have several drink-free days each week. I like to suggest to my clients no drinking between Monday and Thursday.

Summary

The overall message is moderation and hydration! I'm not saying don't drink any alcohol but make sure you're being sensible with your alcohol intake and sticking within the guidelines of 14 units maximum per week. Also, remember to drink 6-8 glasses of water regularly throughout the day to help your body function at its best.

What is a calorie?

Calories can be so misunderstood! At its most basic level, a calorie is a unit of energy. When you see that a food contains 100 calories, that's simply telling you how much energy our bodies could get from eating that food.

Historically, a calorie was defined as the amount of heat needed to raise the temperature of an amount of water by one degree Celsius. When we're talking about food, it's the amount of heat created by burning that food that's needed to cause the one-degree increase in one kilogram of water, which is why you'll see things labelled as kilocalories or kcals. Kilojoules are simply the metric measurement.

How many calories are there in food and drink?

There are four components in food and drink which can be used to generate energy in different amounts when they're broken down by the body during the digestive process. The three main fuel sources are the macronutrients: carbohydrates, protein, and fat. Carbohydrates contain four kcal per gram (they're broken down in around two to three hours into glucose and used to create energy). Protein also contains four kcal per gram (they take about four to five hours to be broken down into amino acids for growth and repair). Fat is the highest, containing nine kcal per gram (taking more than five hours to break down into fatty acids for energy and insulation).

A final component that can yield energy is alcohol, containing seven kcal per gram. Alcohol isn't an optimal fuel source for the body because it doesn't have other nutritional value, but technically it does provide energy.

How much do we need per day?

Our bodies need calories to operate and function. Your body has to have a certain amount of energy to fulfil some of its most basic functions, such as breathing and staying warm. This is your basal metabolic rate or BMR – the rate at which your body uses energy for vital functions during rest. This accounts for about 50-70% of all the energy you use per day.

On top of that, your body requires energy to deal with food, for processes like eating, digesting, using, and storing that food. This can take between 6-10% of your daily energy expenditure. Then there's intentional physical activity. Your body requires energy for planned and unplanned activity, like exercise and moving around. This is highly variable but can take up about 20-40% of your daily energy use.

There's also energy needed for smaller everyday movements like typing, fidgeting, and checking your phone. All these things add up to create your total daily energy expenditure, which needs to be fuelled by energy or calories. Taking in more or less energy than the amount used can lead to either weight gain or weight loss.

Our total daily calorie intake varies hugely from person to person. General guidance on calorie intake by the UK/NHS Eatwell Guide recommends 2,000 calories per day for women and 2,500 for men.

Summary

When thinking about where those calories come from, it is important to remember that both quality and quantity count. These numbers vary hugely, depending on a number of factors including lifestyle, body composition, and activity levels. However, on average, 50% of those calories should come from carbohydrates, 35% from fat, and 15% from protein. For energy, a calorie is a calorie. However, from a health point of view, the nutrients, vitamins, minerals, fibre, sugar, and salt quantities within those foods need to be considered, with the aim of consuming a range of different sources of each macronutrient every day, to provide a truly balanced diet to help your body function as healthily as possible.

Food intolerance

Being intolerant to a number of foods myself, this topic is close to my heart. I want to acknowledge that although a completely balanced diet is ideal, sometimes certain foods have to be avoided or an alternative found. This chapter aims to provide an overview of food intolerances, different types of intolerances, and the distinction between a food intolerance and a food allergy.

Food intolerances are a common occurrence. They appear when the body has difficulty digesting certain food components, leading to uncomfortable symptoms. Some of the most common symptoms are stomach pain, headache, vomiting, and heartburn. While often confused with allergies, food intolerances are different in their underlying causes and manifestations.

"In the UK, an estimated two million people are living with a diagnosed food allergy, and 600,000 with Coeliac Disease". (www.food.gov.uk)

Food Intolerances

Definition and causes

A food intolerance is a non-immune response to a specific food or food component that occurs due to the body's inability to properly digest or process it. The causes of food intolerances can vary, including enzyme deficiencies, sensitivity to additives, chemicals, or natural food components, as well as reactions to certain medications.

Common symptoms

Food intolerances can manifest in various ways, and the symptoms may vary from person to person. Some common symptoms include gastrointestinal issues such as bloating, gas, diarrhoea, or constipation. Additionally, headaches, migraines, skin rashes, fatigue, and mood disturbances can also occur.

Types of Food Intolerances

Lactose intolerance

Lactose intolerance is one of the most prevalent types of food intolerance. It occurs when the body lacks an enzyme known as lactase, which is responsible for breaking down lactose (a sugar found in milk and dairy products). Symptoms can occur soon after consuming lactose-containing products and may range from mild to severe.

Gluten intolerance

Gluten intolerance, also known as non-coeliac gluten sensitivity, is an adverse reaction to gluten – a protein found in wheat, barley, and rye. Unlike coeliac disease, which is an autoimmune disorder, gluten intolerance does not damage the small intestine. Symptoms can include abdominal pain, bloating, diarrhoea, and fatigue.

Fructose malabsorption

Fructose malabsorption is a condition where the small intestine has difficulty absorbing fructose (a sugar found in fruits, honey, and various sweeteners). When consumed in excessive amounts, fructose can lead to gastrointestinal symptoms such as bloating, gas, stomach pain, and diarrhoea.

Food intolerance vs. Food allergy

While food intolerances are non-immune responses, food allergies involve an immune system response to specific food proteins. In food allergies, the body mistakenly identifies harmless food proteins as threats, triggering an immune response that can lead to severe allergic reactions.

Timing and severity of reactions

Food intolerances generally elicit delayed, milder reactions that occur shortly after consuming the triggering food, whereas food allergies tend to have immediate and potentially life-threatening symptoms. Food allergies can cause anaphylaxis, a severe allergic reaction that requires emergency medical attention.

Diagnosis and management

Food intolerances are challenging to diagnose, often requiring food elimination diets or specialised tests. On the other hand, food allergies can be confirmed through skin prick tests, blood tests, or oral food challenges. Both food intolerances and allergies can be managed by avoiding the trigger foods, although food allergies require strict avoidance due to the potential for severe reactions.

Summary

Understanding the differences between food intolerances and allergies is crucial for effectively managing dietary restrictions and ensuring optimal health. While food intolerances can result in discomfort and digestive symptoms, food allergies can be life-threatening. If you suspect you have a food intolerance or allergy, it is essential to consult a healthcare professional for proper diagnosis and guidance on managing your dietary needs.

Top 10 nutrition tips for health

Taking advice from the British Nutrition Foundation and professional experience, below are my top tips to maintain nutritional health and therefore overall happiness and well-being.

1. Maintain a healthy weight

Being overweight or obese is a risk factor for a number of health concerns such as heart disease, stroke, type-2 diabetes, and some cancers, as well as mental health and fertility issues. But what does a healthy weight look like? On a very simplistic and generalised level, knowing your BMI (or Body Mass Index) can be a good starting guide. You can use a BMI calculator on the NHS website which takes into account your height, age, gender, ethnicity, and activity level to categorise your weight and show you where you should aim for. For example, if you are a 6ft 1", 37-year-old male weighing 83kg, you will have a BMI of 23.9. This is within the 'normal' and healthy range for a man of this height, weight, and age. There are lots of ways to maintain a healthy weight and BMI, all of which are covered in various sections of this book.

2. Stay active

Aim for at least 150 minutes each week of moderate-intensity activity, as well as muscle-strengthening exercises for all major muscles. Being physically active every day, even if it's only a short walk, and breaking up long periods of sitting still can also be hugely beneficial.

3. Reduce your red and processed meat intake

On average, if you eat more than 90 grams of red and processed meat a day, it's recommended to try to cut down to 70 grams a day (that's less than 500g per week). Try swapping for leaner and less processed meats and alternative protein sources like eggs, fish, lentils, pulses, and other plant-based alternatives.

4. Eat more fibre

Base your meals on high-fibre and wholegrain foods like wholegrain breakfast cereals, wholewheat pasta, wholemeal bread, brown rice, and pulses like lentils and beans. Unsalted nuts and seeds are also a good source of fibre. These foods will help you feel fuller for longer so you're avoiding the sugary snacks, as well as helping to protect and regulate your insides and help with your digestive and bowel health.

5. Cut down saturated fat

Reduce your intake of processed foods, which can be a high source of saturated fats. Foods like biscuits, cakes, pastries, chocolate, and ready meals can also contain high quantities of salt and sugar. Try unsaturated fats like rapeseed and olive oils, nuts, avocados, and oily fish. Swapping saturated for unsaturated fats and sticking to daily recommended guidelines can have benefits for your heart health as well as your weight!

6. Include more fish in your diet

The UK's Eatwell Guide recommends at least two portions of fish a week, one of which should be oily, like salmon, mackerel, sardines, or trout. If you're a bit unsure of fish, the easiest way to start to get more into your diet is to start with white fish, as this often has a less 'fishy' taste. Experiment with different flavours and ways of preparing it. You can have a look at our recipes section for some ideas.

7. Be careful of salt

High levels of salt in your diet can cause your blood pressure to increase and add extra strain on your heart, increasing your risk of stroke and heart failure. Aim for less than 6g of salt per day. Checking the nutrition label on foods, not adding extra salt to your food, and choosing reduced salt options where possible can help to keep these levels in check.

8. Drink enough water

Drinking water is usually underestimated, but it is absolutely essential for the correct functioning of your body. Try to drink a minimum of 1.5 litres of water per day and more if you are very active or it's a hot day. Other drinks such as squash, juice and hot drinks count, but they are much higher in sugar so try to limit them.

9. Keep track of your alcohol consumption

If you drink alcohol, try not to drink more than 14 units a week, and make sure you're having several alcohol-free days each week as well. These units should be evenly spread across three or more days and binge drinking should be avoided.

10. Ask for help

If you are worried about any aspect of your health, speak to your GP. Other professionals can also help with your nutrition and fitness goals, like a qualified dietitian or a personal trainer.

Eating for happiness

We all know that proper nutrition is essential for our physical health, but did you know that it also plays a significant role in our mental and emotional well-being? In this chapter, we will explore the many ways healthy eating can improve our overall quality of life.

The link between nutrition and mental health

While there are numerous physical benefits of eating a healthy diet, studies from the Mental Health Foundation consistently show that proper nutrition also plays a crucial role in our mental health. Unhealthy diets with high amounts of sugar, processed foods, and saturated fats can increase the risk of depression and anxiety. Conversely, a diet rich in vegetables, fruits, wholegrains, and lean protein has been linked to a lower risk of mental disorders.

Eating for vitality

Eating the right foods can provide the energy and nutrients needed to perform daily activities with ease. Whole foods, such as fruits, vegetables, and wholegrains, provide slow-burning energy, keeping you alert and focused throughout the day.

"Eat regular meals to avoid blood sugar peaks and troughs. Eat a healthy breakfast, space out your meals throughout the day and don't overindulge at one meal. Aim for three small meals with one or two healthy snacks a day." (BBC Food)

The benefits of mindful eating

Mindful eating is the practice of paying attention to your food, your body, and your surroundings while eating. Practising mindful eating can help reduce stress levels and increase the enjoyment of your meals. Additionally, mindful eating can help you tune into your body's signals, such as feeling full or hungry, and avoiding overeating.

Healthy eating and life satisfaction

Eating a healthy diet can also have a profound impact on our overall life satisfaction. When we give our bodies the nutrients and energy they need, we are better able to perform daily activities, engage in physical activity, and maintain positive relationships.

Eating for happiness

Healthy eating can also boost our happiness levels. Foods rich in nutrients like omega-3 fatty acids and antioxidants have been linked to better moods and a lower risk of depression. Additionally, eating foods with vibrant colours and textures can provide visual and sensory pleasure, boosting overall happiness.

Summary

Nourishing yourself through healthy eating can have numerous benefits for your mental, emotional, and physical well-being. Eating a diet rich in whole foods, practising mindful eating, and being consistent in your daily eating habits can lead to an overall improved quality of life, increased energy levels, and greater happiness and satisfaction.

It's not all about lettuce!

I have been saving the most 'yummy' chapter to last! Over the years and forming part of the Live Happy app, the team and I have experimented with nutritionally balanced, tasty and easy recipes that would work for a time-poor, fuss-free person like yourself! All of the following recipes take no more than 30 minutes to make, and all of the macro breakdowns and calories are stated, so if you are tracking your food then this will make it much easier for you. I have chosen the top 25 most popular meals as judged by my clients, but more are available on the Live Happy app. There are veggie, vegan, and pescatarian meals, as well as those for meat eaters, plus advice on how to make some of them gluten or dairy-free if you need to:

Breakfast

Perfect porridge with banana

Oaty banana pancakes

Easy omelette with garlic spinach

Bircher muesli

Eggy breakfast bowl

Lunch

Chopped salad

Pepper and halloumi 4-way wrap

Tahini and mango salad

Tuna with watermelon and feta

Homemade mackerel pâté with crudités

Snacks

Protein banana mug cake

Chewy banana and raisin cookies

Berry cherry smoothie

Mini fruit crumbles

Nutty millionaire's slice

Dinner

Simple sea bass

Orange chicken

Coconut prawns with wild rice

Cod puttanesca

Jackfruit curry

Steak, red cabbage and mash

Chocolate stew

Black bean quesadillas

Honey glazed duck

Stripy fish pie

RECIPES

BREAKFAST

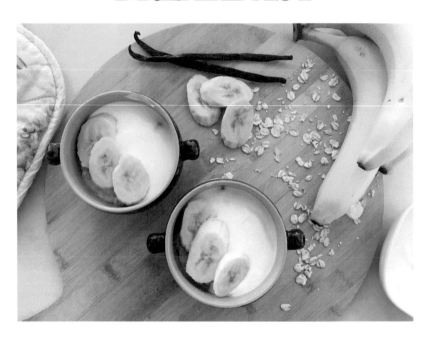

Perfect porridge with banana

Quantity: serves 2

Calories Total (per 1 serving):   206

Calorie Bracket: 200-300

Allergens/Intolerances: GF, Vegan

Fat (g)	6.2
Sat fat (g)	1
Carbs (g)	25.6
Sugar (g)	13.4
Fibre (g)	4.9
Protein (g)	10.3
Salt (g)	0.24

INGREDIENTS

Oatbran	2 tbsp
Jumbo rolled oats	2 tbsp
Unsweetened soya milk	250ml
Soya yoghurt	200g
Banana (peeled, sliced)	1
Vanilla bean paste	2 tsp

METHOD

1. Place oatbran, jumbo oats and soya milk in a small saucepan. Cook for 5 minutes over a medium heat until the oats are tender.

2. Split the cooked oats across two bowls and top each one with half of the soya yoghurt.

3. Share the sliced banana across the two bowls and drizzle each with vanilla paste.

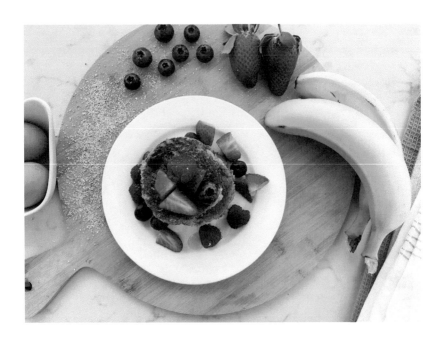

Oaty banana pancakes

Quantity:	serves 2
Calories Total (per 1 serving):	309
Calorie Bracket:	300-400
Allergens/Intolerances:	GF, Vegetarian

Fat (g)	14.2
Sat fat (g)	4.1
Carbs (g)	19.6
Sugar (g)	17.3
Fibre (g)	10.5
Protein (g)	21.1
Salt (g)	0.46

INGREDIENTS

Gluten-free oat flour	1 cup
Egg	1
Banana (peeled, roughly chopped)	1
Unsweetened almond or coconut milk	½ cup
Prune juice	¼ cup
Sea salt	Pinch
Coconut oil	1 tsp

To serve

Berries of your choice	Handful
Maple syrup	¼ cup

METHOD

1. Put all the ingredients and half of the coconut oil into a food processor and blend.

2. Heat the remaining coconut oil in a frying pan over a medium heat.

3. When hot, pour some of the pancake mixture into the pan. Cook the pancakes for a few minutes on each side.

4. Serve hot with berries and maple syrup.

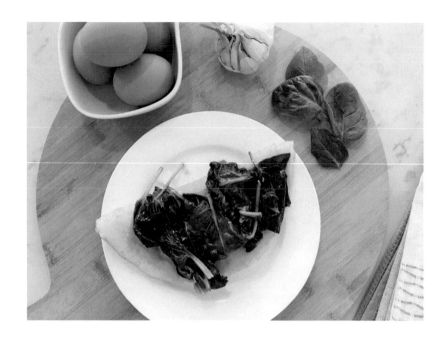

Easy omelette with garlic spinach

Quantity:	serves 2
Calories Total (per 1 serving):	329
Calorie Bracket:	300-400
Allergens/Intolerances:	GF, Vegetarian

Fat (g)	29.6
Sat fat (g)	7.3
Carbs (g)	1.2
Sugar (g)	0.1
Fibre (g)	0.8
Protein (g)	14.4
Salt (g)	0.69

INGREDIENTS

Eggs	4
Rapeseed oil	1 tsp
Unsalted butter or ghee	2 tsp
Olive oil	2 tbsp
Garlic cloves (peeled, minced)	4
Baby spinach	4 cups
Sea salt and black pepper	Pinch

METHOD

1. Crack the eggs into a bowl, whisk and season with salt and pepper.

2. Heat the rapeseed oil and butter in a frying pan over a medium heat until the butter has melted.

3. Pour the eggs into the pan and swirl to cover the surface of the pan completely. Let the mixture cook for about 30 seconds, then flip it over and cook for a further 30 seconds. Remove from the heat and set aside.

4. Heat the olive oil in a frying pan or wok over a medium heat.

5. Add the garlic and cook for 1 minute.

6. Add spinach and season with salt and pepper. Toss the spinach for 1-2 minutes.

7. Remove from heat and serve the garlic spinach on top of the omelette.

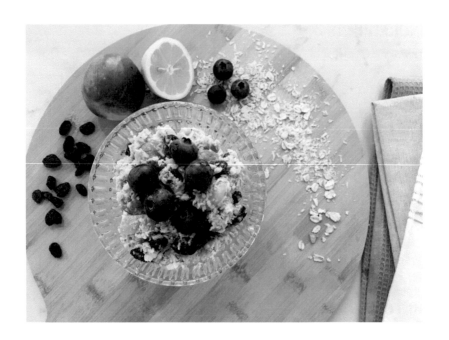

Bircher muesli

Quantity:	serves 2
Calories Total (per 1 serving):	576
Calorie Bracket:	500-600
Allergens/Intolerances:	GF, Vegetarian

Fat (g)	20.3
Sat fat (g)	14.4
Carbs (g)	81.8
Sugar (g)	53
Fibre (g)	12.8
Protein (g)	12.4
Salt (g)	0.26

INGREDIENTS

Jumbo rolled oats	1 cup
Apple (cored, grated)	1
Desiccated coconut	½ cup
Sultanas	½ cup
Dried apricots (chopped)	½ cup
Lemon (juiced)	½
Honey	1 tbsp
Ground cinnamon	½ tsp
Vanilla extract	½ tsp
Unsweetened almond milk	100ml
0% fat Greek yoghurt	3 heaped tbsp

To serve

Blueberries	½ cup

METHOD

1. Place all the ingredients, except the milk and yoghurt, into a mixing bowl and mix together.

2. Add the milk and yoghurt and combine.

3. Leave mixture in the fridge overnight.

4. In the morning, top with berries and enjoy.

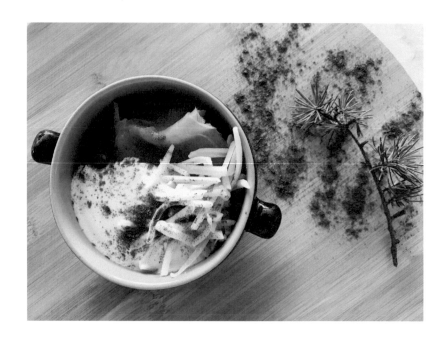

Eggy breakfast bowl

Quantity:	serves 1
Calories Total (per 1 serving):	398
Calorie Bracket:	300-400
Allergens/Intolerances:	GF

Fat (g)	17.5
Sat fat (g)	5.7
Carbs (g)	25.7
Sugar (g)	9.8
Fibre (g)	8.2
Protein (g)	35
Salt (g)	2.9

INGREDIENTS

Eggs	2
Baked beans	150g
Smoked salmon slices	40g
0% fat Greek yoghurt	45g
Paprika	½ tsp
Cheddar cheese (grated)	10g

METHOD

1. Heat a frying pan over a medium heat.

2. Crack the eggs into the pan and continuously stir until they scramble and start to firm up. Remove from the heat.

3. Heat the baked beans in the microwave according to packet instructions (if tinned, remove beans from the tin and place in a bowl before microwaving).

4. Spoon the scrambled eggs into your serving bowl. Add the baked beans.

5. Layer the smoked salmon on top of the beans.

6. Spoon the yoghurt on top of the salmon and sprinkle with paprika.

7. Top with cheese and serve warm.

LUNCH

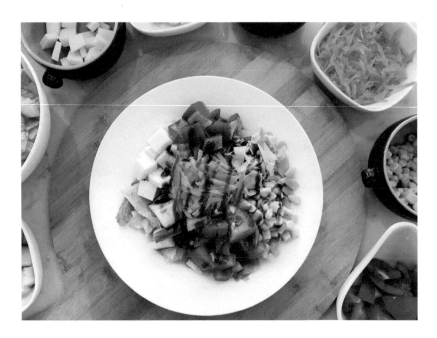

Chopped salad

Quantity:	serves 2
Calories Total (per 1 serving):	394
Calorie Bracket:	300-400
Allergens/Intolerances:	GF

Fat (g)	25.7
Sat fat (g)	9.1
Carbs (g)	21
Sugar (g)	15.3
Fibre (g)	7.5
Protein (g)	18.6
Salt (g)	1.23

INGREDIENTS

Iceberg lettuce (finely chopped)	½
Medium tomatoes (finely chopped)	2
Leerdammer cheese (finely chopped)	70g
Sweetcorn	70g
Wafer thin ham (finely chopped)	5 slices
Cucumber (finely chopped)	¼
Orange pepper (finely chopped)	½
Medium carrot (grated)	1
Extra virgin olive oil	2 tbsp
Balsamic glaze	1 tbsp

METHOD

1. Place the finely chopped ingredients equally into two serving bowls.

2. Drizzle the oil and balsamic glaze over the salad and mix together.

Tip – You can mix up this salad by using your preferred lettuce (like Romaine or Butterhead) and other vegetables you enjoy.

To make this meal vegetarian, swap the ham for a meat-free protein of your choice, like tofu.

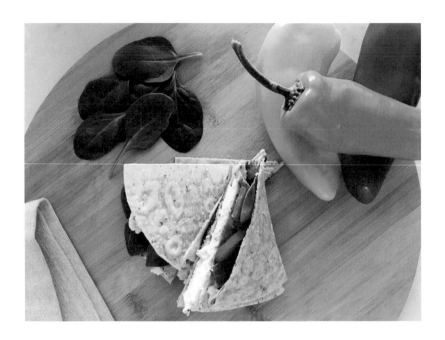

Pepper and halloumi 4-way wrap

Quantity: serves 1
Calories Total (per 1 serving):   594
Calorie Bracket: 500-600
Allergens/Intolerances: Vegetarian

Fat (g)	36.2
Sat fat (g)	11.5
Carbs (g)	44.7
Sugar (g)	5.7
Fibre (g)	6.1
Protein (g)	23.8
Salt (g)	3.3

INGREDIENTS

Olive oil	1 tbsp
Halloumi (thickly sliced)	60g
Red pepper (cored, de-seeded, chopped into large chunks)	½
Flour tortilla or wrap	1
Houmous	50g
Spinach	Handful (25g)

METHOD

1. Heat the oil in a frying pan over a high heat, then add the cheese slices and pepper chunks.

2. Flip the cheese slices over to brown each side and turn the peppers until they soften (approximately 10 minutes).

3. Place the wrap on a chopping board or work surface and make a cut from the centre to one of the edges.

4. Each of the ingredients will be placed on a quarter of the wrap then folded on top of the other to create a triangular pocket. Start with the houmous and spread it evenly over the first quarter near the cut.

5. Place the cooked halloumi onto the second quarter and fold the houmous quarter over it.

6. Place the peppers in the third quarter and fold the houmous/halloumi section over it.

7. Place the spinach on the final quarter and fold over to create the triangular pocket with all the quarters layered together.

8. Cut the pocket in half to make it easier to eat. Enjoy hot or cold.

Tip – Once the pocket has been constructed, you can toast both sides in a hot pan to warm the sandwich through.

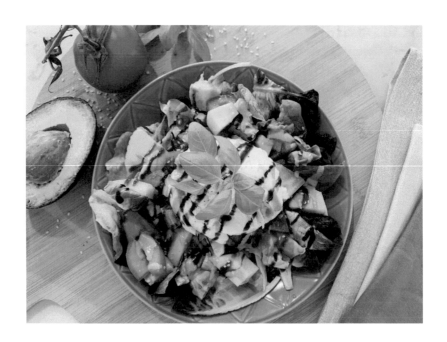

Tahini and mango salad

Quantity:	serves 1
Calories Total (per 1 serving):	819
Calorie Bracket:	800-900
Allergens/Intolerances:	GF

Fat (g)	59.6
Sat fat (g)	22.2
Carbs (g)	41.2
Sugar (g)	38.5
Fibre (g)	9.6
Protein (g)	29.6
Salt (g)	1.62

INGREDIENTS

Butterhead salad leaves (roughly chopped)	1 large handful
Tomato (cubed)	1
Avocado (peeled, de-stoned, cubed)	1
Mango (peeled, de-stoned, cubed)	1
Tahini	2 tbsp
Balsamic glaze	1 tsp
Lemon juice	1 tsp
Mozzarella	1 ball
Fresh basil	1 small handful
Sea salt and black pepper	Pinch
Sesame seeds	Pinch

METHOD

1. Place the salad leaves on a serving plate or bowl and add the tomato, avocado and the mango cubes.

2. Place the mozzarella ball in the centre of the salad and add the basil leaves.

3. Drizzle the tahini, balsamic glaze and lemon across the salad and add a pinch of salt, pepper and sesame seeds over the top.

4. Sprinkle the fresh basil leaves over the salad

5. Serve immediately as a vegetarian lunch or add grilled chicken for extra protein.

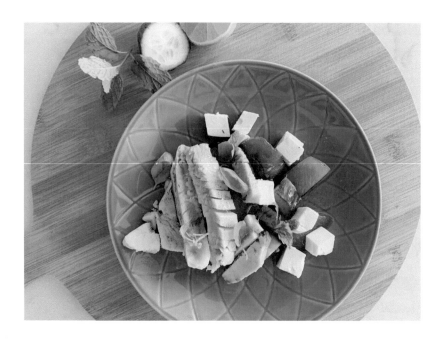

Tuna with watermelon and feta

Quantity: serves 2
Calories Total (per 1 serving):   297
Calorie Bracket: 200-300
Allergens/Intolerances: GF

Fat (g)	11
Sat fat (g)	23.4
Carbs (g)	11.5
Sugar (g)	11.45
Fibre (g)	0.55
Protein (g)	38.9
Salt (g)	1.1

INGREDIENTS

Tuna steak	250g
Olive oil	Drizzle
Watermelon (chunks)	200g
Feta	75g
Lime	½
Fresh basil, mint	Half handful
Cucumber	½
Honey	8g

METHOD

1. Preheat the frying pan and rub the tuna steak in oil and add salt. Cook steak on each side.

2. Place the tuna steak on a plate to rest.

3. Place the watermelon, feta, cucumber, mint and basil leaves to a mixing bowl and gently stir the mix.

4. Add salt and pepper and add entire mixture on the plate next to the tuna.

5. Add honey, lime juice, olive oil and salt.

6. Stir and add to the watermelon mixture on the plate.

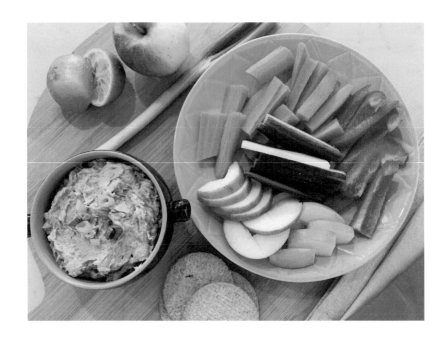

Homemade mackerel pâté with crudités

Quantity:	serves 2
Calories Total (per 1 serving):	555
Calorie Bracket:	500-600
Allergens/Intolerances:	Dairy-free, GF

Fat (g)	33.2
Sat fat (g)	9.25
Carbs (g)	36.4
Sugar (g)	16.9
Fibre (g)	7.1
Protein (g)	27.3
Salt (g)	4.7

INGREDIENTS

Smoked mackerel fillets (skin and bones removed)	200g
Lime (zested, juiced)	1
Fresh ginger	4 cm
Dairy-free coconut yoghurt	4 tbsp
Gluten-free soy sauce	2 tbsp
Spring onions	4
Sea salt and black pepper	Pinch

To serve:

Apple (cored, sliced)	1
Red pepper (de-seeded, sliced)	1
Carrot (sliced)	1
Cucumber (sliced)	1
Gluten-free oat cakes	6

METHOD

1. Place all the ingredients in a food processor or blender and mix until combined well.

2. Taste and season accordingly.

3. Spoon the pâté into bowls and serve with the oat cakes, sliced apple and vegetables on the side. Enjoy!

Tip – You can use 2 tablespoons of organic mayonnaise instead of the dairy-free coconut yoghurt if preferred.

SNACKS

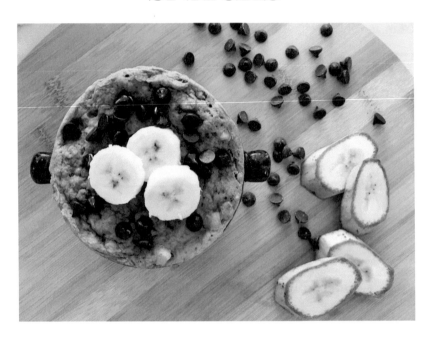

Protein banana mug cake

Quantity:	serves 1
Calories Total (per 1 serving):	303
Calorie Bracket:	300-400
Allergens/Intolerances:	Vegetarian

Fat (g)	6
Sat fat (g)	3.6
Carbs (g)	39.7
Sugar (g)	26.8
Fibre (g)	1.9
Protein (g)	24
Salt (g)	0.31

INGREDIENTS

Banana (peeled, mashed)	½
Self-raising flour	2 tbsp
Protein powder	1 scoop (25g)
Baking powder	½ tsp
Maple syrup	1 tbsp
Unsweetened almond milk (or milk of any kind)	2 tbsp
Chocolate chips	1 tbsp

METHOD

1. In a microwave proof mug, add all the ingredients and mix thoroughly.

2. Microwave (800w) for 90 seconds.

3. Enjoy hot.

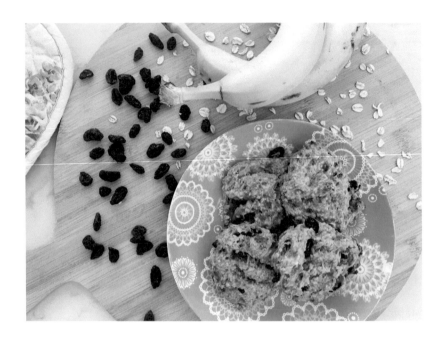

Chewy banana and raisin cookies

Quantity:	serves 6
Calories Total (per 1 serving):	231
Calorie Bracket:	200-300
Allergens/Intolerances:	Vegan

Fat (g)	10.7
Sat fat (g)	8.2
Carbs (g)	32.5
Sugar (g)	17.1
Fibre (g)	2.3
Protein (g)	3
Salt (g)	0.43

INGREDIENTS

Bananas (peeled, mashed)	2
Rolled oats	1 cup
Spelt or plain flour	¼ cup
Raisins	½ cup
Maple syrup	1 tbsp
Unrefined coconut oil (melted)	¼ cup
Vanilla essence or paste	1 tsp
Ground allspice (or ground cinnamon)	1½ tsp
Sea salt	½ tsp

METHOD

1. Preheat the oven to 170°C (fan assisted).

2. Line a large baking tray with parchment/baking paper.

3. Place all the ingredients in a large bowl. Stir until everything is evenly combined.

4. Using a tablespoon, scoop up some mixture and drop it onto the baking paper. Using the back of the spoon, flatten slightly into a cookie shape.

5. Repeat, spacing the cookie dough about 3 inches apart.

6. Bake for 18-20 minutes or until the edges of the cookies are golden brown. Leave to cool and enjoy!

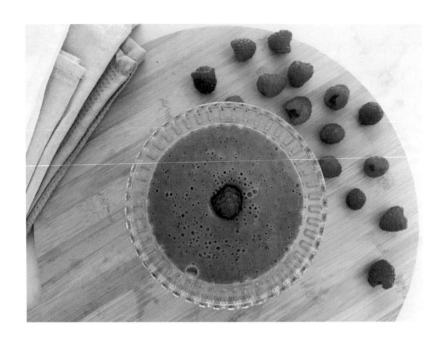

Berry cherry smoothie

Quantity:	serves 1
Calories Total (per 1 serving):	91
Calorie Bracket:	under 100
Allergens/Intolerances:	GF, Vegetarian

Fat (g)	0.6
Sat fat (g)	0.3
Carbs (g)	14.3
Sugar (g)	13.8
Fibre (g)	3.8
Protein (g)	6.7
Salt (g)	0.16

INGREDIENTS

0% fat Greek yoghurt	50g
Skimmed milk	50ml
Water	50ml
Fresh or frozen raspberries	50g
Frozen cherries	50g

METHOD

1. Place all the ingredients in a blender and process until completely smooth.

2. Best enjoyed immediately.

Tip – To make this recipe vegan, use plant-based products like almond milk and soya yoghurt.

You can add ice to give your smoothie a thick, chilly texture.

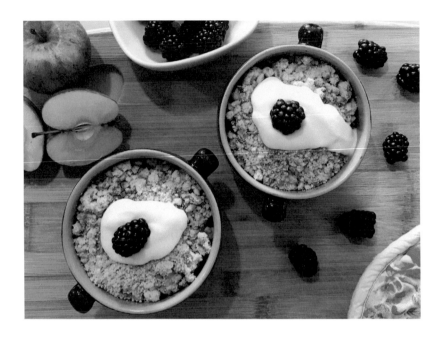

Mini fruit crumbles

Quantity:	serves 2
Calories Total (per 1 serving):	499
Calorie Bracket:	400-500
Allergens/Intolerances:	Vegetarian

Fat (g)	29.9
Sat fat (g)	14.2
Carbs (g)	46.8
Sugar (g)	20.9
Fibre (g)	5.7
Protein (g)	9.6
Salt (g)	0.11

INGREDIENTS

Apples (cored, diced)	2
Water	50ml
Maple syrup	1 tbsp
Blackberries	60g
Ground almonds	20g
Ground cinnamon	1 tsp
Plain flour	60g
Pre-made granola	20g
Unsalted butter (melted)	50g
0% fat Greek yoghurt	2 tbsp

METHOD

1. Preheat the oven to 180°C (fan assisted).

2. Place the apples in a pan with the water. Bring to the boil, then reduce to a simmer for 10 minutes to soften the apples.

3. Add the maple syrup and blackberries and simmer for a further 2 minutes.

4. Transfer the fruit mixture into two small oven proof dishes.

5. Place the ground almonds, cinnamon, flour, granola and butter in a mixing bowl. Stir until small clumps of mixture start to form.

6. Add the crumble mixture to the top of the fruit and bake in the oven for 12-15 minutes, until the tops start to brown.

7. Remove from the oven and leave to cool for a few minutes before topping with Greek yoghurt to serve.

Tip – These are also nice served cold the next morning for breakfast.

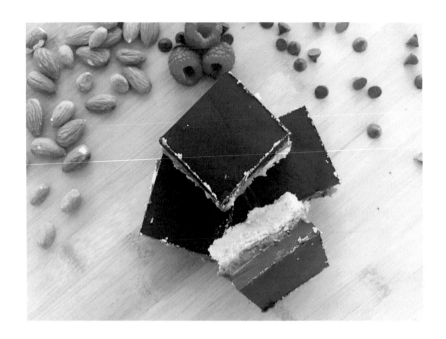

Nutty millionaire's slice

Quantity:	serves 14
Calories Total (per 1 serving):	301
Calorie Bracket:	300-400
Allergens/Intolerances:	Vegetarian

Fat (g)	25.9
Sat fat (g)	8.3
Carbs (g)	8.7
Sugar (g)	2.7
Fibre (g)	4.8
Protein (g)	8.2
Salt (g)	0.09

INGREDIENTS

Ground almonds	150g
Plain flour	50g
Unsalted butter (melted)	70g
Coconut oil	20g
Peanut butter	100g
Almond butter	100g
Maple syrup	2 tbsp
Whole almonds	50g
Low-sugar dark chocolate (melted)	160g

METHOD

1. Preheat the oven to 170°C (fan assisted).
2. **Layer 1 (base):** In a mixing bowl, combine the ground almonds, flour, melted butter and half of the coconut oil until it stiffens into a crumbly dough.
3. Line an oven proof dish with greaseproof paper. Spread and pat down the base mixture so that it covers the base of the dish in a layer 1cm thick.
4. Bake in the oven for 20 minutes, until the top just starts to brown.
5. Leave to cool before adding the next layer.
6. **Layer 2 (filling):** In a mixing bowl, combine the peanut butter, almond butter, maple syrup and whole almonds.
7. Spread the mixture evenly over layer 1 and place in the fridge to harden slightly, whilst you prepare the final layer.
8. **Layer 3 (topping):** Mix the remaining coconut oil into the melted chocolate.
9. Pour the chocolate mixture evenly over layer 2.
10. Place the whole dish in the fridge to set. This is best left overnight but needs an hour minimum.
11. When ready to serve, remove from the dish, remove the greaseproof paper and slice into squares.

Tip – Slices are best kept in the fridge until ready to consume.

DINNER

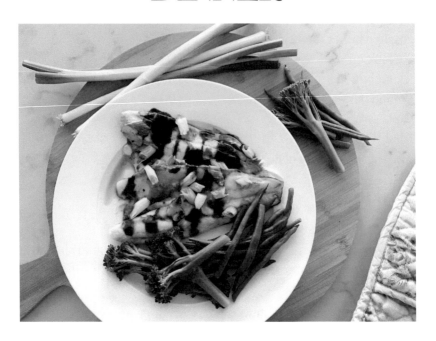

Simple sea bass

Quantity:	serves 2
Calories Total (per 1 serving):	273
Calorie Bracket:	200-300
Allergens/Intolerances:	GF

Fat (g)	16.1
Sat fat (g)	3
Carbs (g)	9.3
Sugar (g)	6,7
Fibre (g)	5.8
Protein (g)	22.8
Salt (g)	2.11

INGREDIENTS

Sea bass fillets	2
Gluten-free soy sauce	1 tbsp
Sesame oil	1 tbsp
White wine vinegar	1 tbsp
Gluten-free oyster sauce	2 tbsp
Spring onions (sliced)	2
Broccoli (cut into small florets)	1 (medium)
Green beans (trimmed)	Handful

METHOD

1. Preheat the oven to 180°C (fan assisted).

2. Place the sea bass, skin down, in an oven proof dish.

3. Pour the soy sauce, sesame oil, white wine vinegar and oyster sauce over the top of the fish, then sprinkle over the spring onion pieces.

4. Bake in the oven for 20 minutes.

5. Bring a pan of water to the boil and cook the broccoli and green beans until tender.

6. Remove the fish from the oven. Place gently on a plate and serve with the vegetables.

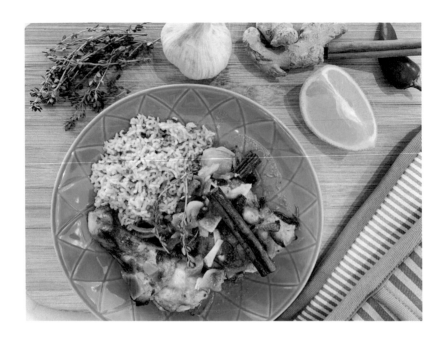

Orange chicken

Quantity:	serves 2
Calories Total (per 1 serving):	564
Calorie Bracket:	500-600
Allergens/Intolerances:	GF

Fat (g)	38
Sat fat (g)	9.7
Carbs (g)	19.8
Sugar (g)	16.5
Fibre (g)	3.5
Protein (g)	34.4
Salt (g)	0.56

INGREDIENTS

Olive oil	2 tbsp
Chicken thighs and drumsticks	4
Medium orange (juiced, peel grated)	1
Red onion (peeled, diced)	1
Garlic paste	2 tsp
Ginger (finely grated)	5cm
Red wine vinegar	2 tbsp
Clear honey	2 tbsp
Cinnamon stick	2
Fresh thyme sprigs	4
Saffron strands	½ tsp (optional)

METHOD

1. Preheat the oven to $200°C$ (fan assisted).

2. Mix all the ingredients in a bowl, rubbing everything into the chicken.

3. Place the chicken pieces onto a roasting tray. Bake uncovered for 30 minutes.

4. Check the chicken is fully cooked by testing the thickest part with a fork to make sure the juices run clear before serving.

Tip – Serve with fluffy couscous or white rice.

Add ½ tsp of saffron to spice it up.

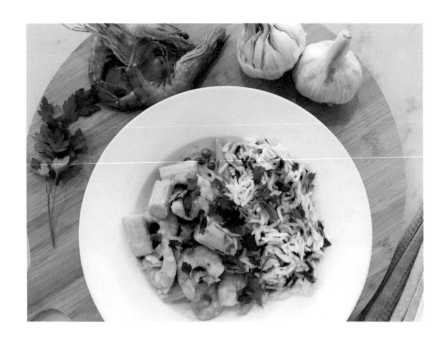

Coconut prawns with wild rice

Quantity:	serves 2
Calories Total (per 1 serving):	676
Calorie Bracket:	600-700
Allergens/Intolerances:	Dairy-free, GF

Fat (g)	32.6
Sat fat (g)	26.7
Carbs (g)	65.4
Sugar (g)	11.9
Fibre (g)	9.9
Protein (g)	33.6
Salt (g)	0.74

INGREDIENTS

Wild rice	60g
Brown basmati rice	60g
Coconut oil	2 tbsp
White onion (peeled, diced)	1
Baby corn (chopped)	200g
Fresh or frozen peas	100g
Garlic cloves (peeled, minced)	2
Ground turmeric	1 tsp
Tin of coconut milk	½ (200ml)
Raw tiger prawns	225g
Fresh parsley (chopped)	Handful

METHOD

1. Cook both rices in separate pans according to the instructions on the packet.

2. Heat the oil in a frying pan or wok over a medium heat. Sauté the onion for 5 minutes.

3. Add the corn, peas, garlic and turmeric and sauté for a further 3 minutes.

4. Add the coconut milk and bring to the boil, then reduce the heat and simmer for 6 minutes.

5. Add the prawns and simmer for a further 5 minutes.

6. Serve with the rice and a sprinkle of parsley.

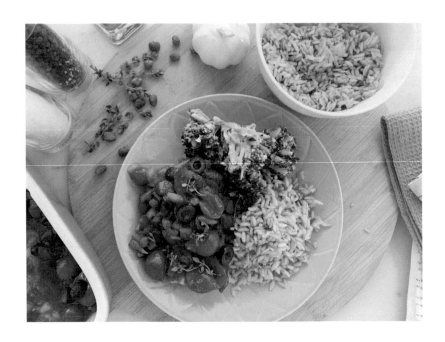

Cod puttanesca

Quantity:	serves 2
Calories Total (per 1 serving):	300
Calorie Bracket:	300-400
Allergens/Intolerances:	Dairy-free, GF

Fat (g)	11.85
Sat fat (g)	1.75
Carbs (g)	27.4
Sugar (g)	2.45
Fibre (g)	3.3
Protein (g)	18.4
Salt (g)	2.4

INGREDIENTS

Skinless and boneless cod fillets	250g
Olive oil	1 tbsp
Onion (peeled, chopped)	1
Garlic clove (peeled, crushed)	1
Anchovies (drained, chopped)	5 (optional)
Tin of cherry tomatoes	1
Capers (rinsed)	2 tbsp
Pitted black olives (halved)	40g
Thyme sprigs (leaves only, stalks removed)	2

To serve:

Extra virgin olive oil	Drizzle
Brown rice	100g
Broccoli (cut into florets)	2 handfuls

METHOD

1. Preheat the oven to 170°C (fan assisted).
2. Cook the rice according to packet instructions.
3. Heat the oil in a frying pan over a medium heat and add the onion, garlic and the anchovies. Cook for about 6-8 minutes or until softened.
4. Add the cherry tomatoes, capers, olives, thyme and a little seasoning then lower heat and simmer for 5 minutes.
5. Transfer the sauce to a small oven proof dish.
6. Add the cod to the dish, ensuring the cod fillets are nestled in the sauce and bake for 12-15 minutes until the fish is opaque and flaky.
7. While the cod is cooking, boil or steam the broccoli florets.
8. Drizzle the fish with a little olive oil to serve, splitting over two bowls with the rice and broccoli.

Tip – This puttanesca works well served on its own with some crusty bread or with wholemeal pasta instead of rice.

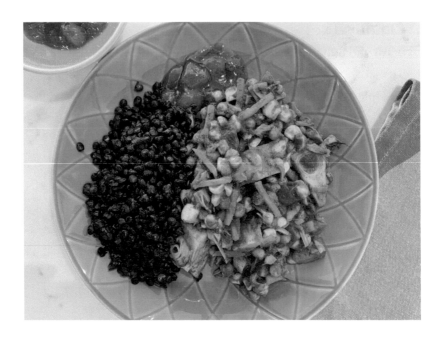

Jackfruit curry

Quantity:	serves 2
Calories Total (per 1 serving):	439
Calorie Bracket:	400-500
Allergens/Intolerances:	GF, Vegetarian

Fat (g)	11.2
Sat fat (g)	1.3
Carbs (g)	54.5
Sugar (g)	17.8
Fibre (g)	23.6
Protein (g)	22.7
Salt (g)	1.46

INGREDIENTS

Olive oil	1 tsp
White onion (peeled, diced)	1
Tin of jackfruit (drained, rinsed)	1
Tikka masala spice paste	3 tbsp
Tomato passata	200g
Fresh or frozen mixed vegetables (finely chopped)	350g
Mango chutney	2 tbsp
Puy lentils (pre-cooked microwave packet)	1 packet (250g)

METHOD

1. Heat the oil in a frying pan over a medium heat.

2. Add the onions and cook for 5 minutes until softened.

3. Break up the jackfruit into the pan and cook for about 10 minutes, stirring occasionally.

4. Mix in the spice paste and passata.

5. Add the mixed vegetables and stir everything together, ensuring it is well combined. Cook for a further 10 minutes, stirring occasionally.

6. Add 1 tbsp of mango chutney and stir through.

7. Cook the puy lentils according to packet instructions.

8. Serve the curry mixture with the puy lentils and the remaining mango chutney.

Tip – Depending on your preferences, jackfruit can be swapped for chicken or lamb, and the lentils for rice.

You can use another flavour of spice paste to make this recipe milder or hotter.

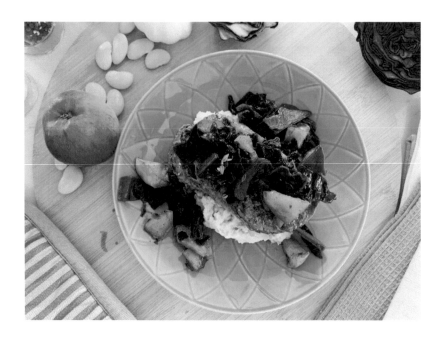

Steak, red cabbage and mash

Quantity:	serves 2
Calories Total (per 1 serving):	807
Calorie Bracket:	800-900
Allergens/Intolerances:	GF

Fat (g)	26
Sat fat (g)	14.3
Carbs (g)	102.3
Sugar (g)	25.6
Fibre (g)	16.3
Protein (g)	44.9
Salt (g)	0.37

INGREDIENTS

Large potatoes (chopped)	2
Apple (peeled, cored, sliced)	1
Ground cinnamon	½ tsp
Honey	2 tbsp
Red cabbage (sliced)	90g
Tin of butter beans (drained, rinsed)	1
Garlic clove (peeled, crushed)	2
Unsalted butter	40g
Fillet or sirloin steak	200g
Wholegrain mustard	1 tbsp
Fresh thyme	2 sprigs

METHOD

1. Place a pan of water on a high heat and, once boiling, add in the potatoes for approximately 15 minutes until very soft.

2. Whilst the potatoes are boiling, place the apple slices in a separate pan on a medium heat. Add the honey and cinnamon and soften the apple slices.

3. Place the red cabbage into a pan of water and boil for a few minutes until soft.

4. Add the cooked red cabbage to the apple mixture and stir in gently.

5. Put the butter beans, half the butter and garlic in a blender and blend until smooth.

6. Strain the cooked potatoes and mash until smooth.

7. Add the butter bean mixture to the mashed potatoes and reheat.

8. Place the remaining butter in a frying pan on a high heat. Fry the steaks to your liking. Once the steaks are nearly cooked, add the mustard and thyme and coat the steaks.

9. Place the mash and red cabbage mixture on your plate and top with the steak. Sprinkle a little more thyme on the top and serve immediately.

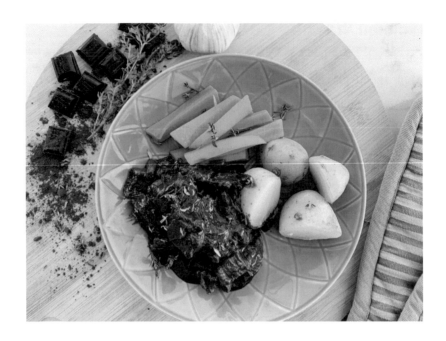

Chocolate stew

Quantity:	serves 2
Calories Total (per 1 serving):	556
Calorie Bracket:	500-600
Allergens/Intolerances:	GF

Fat (g)	25.6
Sat fat (g)	9
Carbs (g)	26.9
Sugar (g)	11.25
Fibre (g)	8.5
Protein (g)	53.6
Salt (g)	0.3

INGREDIENTS

Olive oil	1 tbsp
Red onion (peeled, finely diced)	1
Garlic cloves (peeled, crushed)	2
Beef brisket (diced)	300g
New potatoes	6 medium
Carrots (chopped)	2 large
Chipotle paste	½ tsp
Smoked paprika	1 tsp
Tomato purée	4 tbsp
Beef stock cube	1
Cacao powder	1 tbsp
Fresh thyme	2-3 sprigs

METHOD

1. Heat the oil in a large pan over a high heat and add the onion and garlic. Add in the beef and keep stirring until the beef is browned.

2. In a separate pan, boil some water and cook the new potatoes for about 15 minutes until soft but not falling apart. Add the carrots about halfway through the process.

3. Whilst the potatoes and carrots are cooking, stir in the chipotle paste, paprika and tomato purée to the beef.

4. Mix up the beef stock according to packet instructions and add to the pan. Finally, add the cacao powder and stir everything together. Simmer until the vegetables are cooked.

5. Plate up the beef stew with the vegetables and sprinkle the thyme over the top. Serve immediately.

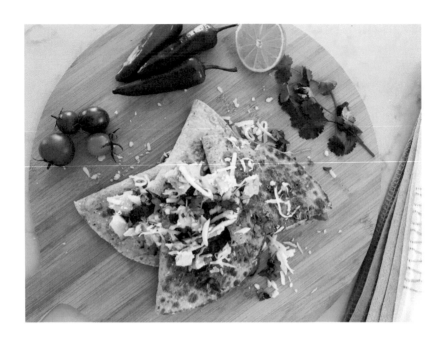

Black bean quesadillas

Quantity: serves 4
Calories Total (per 1 serving): 603
Calorie Bracket: 600-700
Allergens/Intolerances: Vegetarian

Fat (g)	31.8
Sat fat (g)	14.2
Carbs (g)	51.3
Sugar (g)	8.5
Fibre (g)	10.3
Protein (g)	24.9
Salt (g)	1.65

INGREDIENTS

Olive oil	1 tbsp
White onion (peeled, diced)	½
Tin of sweetcorn (drained, rinsed)	1 (200g)
Tin of black beans (drained, rinsed)	1 (400g)
Cherry tomatoes (quartered)	250g
Fresh chilli (de-seeded, finely chopped)	1 (small)
Ground cumin	1 tbsp
Lime (juiced)	1
Sea salt	Pinch
Fresh coriander (chopped)	Small bunch
Flour tortillas or wraps	4
Cheddar cheese (grated)	200g
Avocado (peeled, de-stoned, thinly sliced)	1

METHOD

1. Heat the oil in a frying pan over a high heat.
2. Add the onion and sweetcorn and cook for a few minutes until they start to brown.
3. Add the black beans, cherry tomatoes, chilli, cumin, juice from half the lime and salt. Stir for a few minutes until combined and heated through. Take off the heat and put the mixture in a bowl.
4. Stir half of the coriander into the vegetable mixture and set aside.
5. Heat a dry frying pan over a medium heat.
6. Place a tortilla in the frying pan. On one half of the tortilla, add a generous handful of cheese, a few spoonfuls of the vegetable mix and another handful of cheese.
7. Fold the plain half of the tortilla over the mixture half and push together. When the tortilla has browned and the cheese has started to melt, carefully flip it over to toast the other side.
8. Repeat for remaining tortillas.
9. Serve with a sprinkle of coriander and avocado, and add the rest of the lime juice over the top.

Tip – To make this recipe vegan, substitute the cheese for a dairy-free alternative. To add some meat, fry chicken pieces with a Mexican spice mix and add to the tortilla alongside the cheese and vegetables.

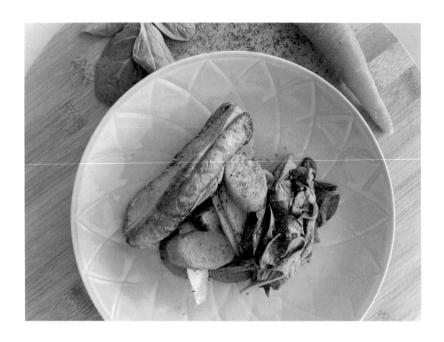

Honey glazed duck

Quantity:	serves 1
Calories Total (per 1 serving):	479
Calorie Bracket:	400-500
Allergens/Intolerances:	Dairy-free, GF

Fat (g)	18.1
Sat fat (g)	4.4
Carbs (g)	52.7
Sugar (g)	39.1
Fibre (g)	8.7
Protein (g)	30.1
Salt (g)	0.54

INGREDIENTS

Duck breast	1
Honey	2 tbsp
Carrots (chopped)	2
Dried basil	1 tsp
Oregano	1 tsp
Onion powder	1 tsp
Garlic powder	1 tsp
Olive oil	Drizzle
Parsnip (chopped)	1 large
Spinach	2 handfuls

METHOD

1. Score the duck breast. Place skin side down and shallow fry for 2 minutes each side.

2. Place the duck in the oven at 180°C for 10 minutes.

3. Chop the carrots and parsnips into small chunks and add a drizzle of olive oil.

4. Next, add the dried basil, oregano and onion powder. Cook in the oven for 15 minutes

5. Once you've taken out the duck, gently brush honey on to the scored side of the duck breast, and let it cool until time to plate.

6. In a small saucepan, add spinach and garlic powder. Cook on medium/low for 2 minutes and take out just before its wilted.

7. Plate the food and drizzle honey over the carrots and parsnips.

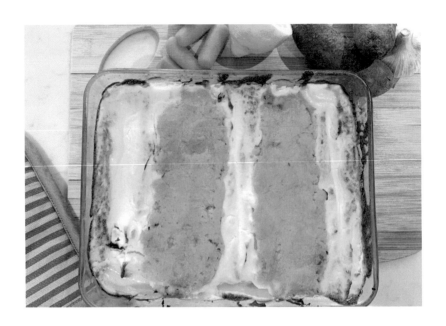

Stripy fish pie

Quantity:	serves 6-8
Calories Total (per 1 serving):	365
Calorie Bracket:	300-400
Allergens/Intolerances:	GF

Fat (g)	18.6
Sat fat (g)	6.8
Carbs (g)	20.5
Sugar (g)	8.3
Fibre (g)	4.9
Protein (g)	30.4
Salt (g)	1.57

INGREDIENTS

Salmon fillets (skin removed, bite-sized chunks)	300g
Undyed smoked haddock fillets (skin removed, bite-sized chunks)	300g
Raw king prawns (peeled)	125g
Lemon (juiced)	1
Olive oil	1 tbsp
Sea salt	Large pinch
Black pepper	Large pinch
Carrots (peeled, finely diced)	2
Celery stalks (finely diced)	2
Fresh flat leaf parsley sprigs (finely chopped)	4

Topping:

Sweet potatoes (peeled, chopped)	2 large
Large cauliflower (green leaves removed, chopped)	1
Garlic cloves (peeled)	2
Unsalted butter (optional)	1 tbsp
Cheddar cheese (grated)	100g (optional)
Sea salt	Large pinch
Black pepper	Large pinch

METHOD

1. Preheat the oven to 200°C (fan assisted) and heat two saucepans of water.

2. Place the salmon, smoked haddock and prawns into an oven proof baking dish.

3. Squeeze the lemon juice over the baking dish. Add the olive oil and season with salt and pepper.

4. Add the carrots, celery and parsley and mix everything together well. Set the dish aside and prepare the topping.

5. When one saucepan of water is boiling, add the sweet potato and cook until soft.

6. In the second saucepan, boil the cauliflower and garlic with the lid on for 5 minutes or until the cauliflower is tender (use a knife to check).

7. Drain the cauliflower, add the butter and cheese (optional) and the salt and pepper. Blend or mash until creamy and smooth.

8. When the sweet potato is ready, drain and blend or mash until smooth.

9. Layer the cauliflower mash and the sweet potato in strips on top of the fish mixture with the back of a fork, until the dish is evenly covered in a stripy pattern.

10. Bake in the oven for 25 minutes, or until cooked through with a crispy, golden top. Serve piping hot.

Tip – Most supermarkets have a fresh fish counter and will fillet and cut the fish into chunks for you.

Alternatively, look for a pack of assorted fish and shellfish for pie filling – you'll want about 700-750g for this recipe.

EPILOGUE: ON BALANCE...

Thank you for sticking with me throughout this happiness roller-coaster ride! Together, we have peeled back the layers of the complexity of happiness and unveiled the scientific truth behind why we feel and react the way we do. We have summarised the activities and types of people that bring us joy and happiness, and how to do more of the things that give us these positive feelings. We have also touched on the sad moments in life and acknowledged this is part of the journey of life as well. If you have completed the Action Time activities at the end of each chapter in the Feel section, then this will give you a blueprint to guide you to a happier life.

I hope you agree I have been honest with you throughout the whole journey of this book. Here's another truth: Don't be naive enough to think you can float through life and everything will be perfect and amazing all the time. Shit happens and sometimes it's very difficult to remain positive and happy. But strive to find balance in your life and it will generally work out for you. Balance is the key!

"Three grand essentials to happiness in this life are; something to do, something to love and something to hope for."

Joseph Addison (1672 – 1719)
English poet and politician

Here is my summary of trying to find happiness, based on scientific research, my life experience, and my job:

- Eat healthily but enjoy your food.

- Exercise regularly, but not to the extreme where you are constantly experiencing Delayed Onset Muscle Soreness (DOMS) all the time and getting injured.

- Look after your mind without feeling like you have to be in a constant state of zen all day.

- Make some decent friends.

- Get a dog and take it for a walk every day.

- Try not to drink too much alcohol.

- Have something positive to say about others – fill their 'cup' as opposed to draining it.

- Try to find some joy in your job, as you spend a lot of time there – if you absolutely hate it, quit and do something you really want to do, even if the money isn't as good.

- Pots of money does not necessarily bring you happiness, but having enough to pay your way, taking a holiday at least once a year, and not worrying about the mortgage bouncing each month, is perfect!

"To be kind to all, to like many and love a few,
to be needed and wanted by those we love,
is certainly the nearest we can come to happiness."

Mary Stuart (1542 – 1567)
Queen of Scots

My philosophy on life is that we aren't on this planet for that long, so make the most of it as opposed to thinking "I could have done more," or "I wish I had worried less". Read this book, soak in as much as you can, and try to do as many things as you can that make you personally happy. Write a list and get cracking through it!

When I visited the Delphin Be Grand Hotel in Antalya, Turkey, recently, I was reminded every morning and evening by these words, beautifully designed around the outside of their bathroom mirrors:

"Be kind, be nice, be positive, be amazing, be happy."

REFERENCES

INTRO:

The Happiness Project, Body Worlds Museum, Amsterdam
www.bodyworlds.nl/en/

Section 1: FEEL

1A – Defining Happiness

What is Happiness?

Sonja Lyubomirsky, *The How of Happiness*, Piatkus, 2010
https://greatergood.berkeley.edu/topic/happiness/definition

Kendra Cherry
www.verywellmind.com/what-is-happiness-4869755

Aristotle, *Nicomachean Ethics*, Penguin, 2020
www.thepursuitofhappiness.org

Steven Greer & Maggie Watson, 'Mental adjustment to cancer: its measurement and prognostic importance', *Cancer Surveys 1987*, Vol. 6, No. 3, (1987)

Harvard University Study of Adult Development
www.adultdevelopmentstudy.org

Vibeke Koushede, contributor, *The Future of Wellbeing in an Ageing Society*, Happiness Research Institute, 2022

Corporate Finance Institute
https://corporatefinanceinstitute.com/resources/career-map/sell-side/capital-markets/hedonic-treadmill/

Grant E Donnelly, Tianyi Zeng, Emily Haisley & Michael I Norton, *The Happiness of Millionaires*, Harvard Business School
www.hbs.edu/faculty/Pages/item.aspx?num=53540

The Happiness Project, Body Worlds Museum, Amsterdam
www.bodyworlds.nl/en/

Dr Marianna Pogosyan, *How Genes Influence Happiness*, 2019
www.psychologytoday.com/us/blog/between-cultures/201911/how-genes-influence-happiness

The Happiness Project, Body Worlds Museum, Amsterdam
www.bodyworlds.nl/en/

Balancing the Triangle of Life

Harvard University Study of Adult Development
www.adultdevelopmentstudy.org

Paul Richlovsky, *Is a Balanced Work-Life Relationship Overrated?*
www.topresume.com/career-advice/is-a-balanced-work-life-relationship-overrated

Cultivating Gratitude

The Science of Gratitude
www.mindful.org/the-science-of-gratitude/

Giving Thanks Can Make You Happier
www.health.harvard.edu/healthbeat/giving-thanks-can-make-you-happier

How to Practice Gratitude
www.mindful.org/an-introduction-to-mindful-gratitude/

The Science of Kindness
www.randomactsofkindness.org/the-science-of-kindness

R McCraty, B Barrios-Choplin, D Rozman, M Atkinson & A D Watkins, 'The impact of a new emotional self-management program on stress, emotions, heart rate variability, DHEA and cortisol', *Integrative physiological and behavioral science : the official journal of the Pavlovian Society,* 1998 Apr-Jun, 33(2), pp151-70.
https://pubmed.ncbi.nlm.nih.gov/9737736/

Watch Out – Happiness is Catching!

The Happiness Project, Body Worlds Museum, Amsterdam
www.bodyworlds.nl/en/

N.A. Christakis, Framingham Heart Study, Harvard, (2008), *BMJ* 2008, 337, a2338
https://doi.org/10.1136/bmj.a2338

Yoram Barak, 'The Immune System and Happiness', *Autoimmunity Reviews*, 2006, Vol. 5, Issue 8, pp 523-527
www.sciencedirect.com/science/article/abs/pii/S1568997206000279

The Power of Laughter

The Happiness Project, Body Worlds Museum, Amsterdam
www.bodyworlds.nl/en/

Betty-Anne Heggie, 'The Healing Power of Laughter', *Journal of Hospital Medicine*, 2019 May; 14(5): 320.
www.ncbi.nlm.nih.gov/pmc/articles/PMC6609137/

Blackadder the Third, Episode 2, 'Ink and Incapability', BBC TV, 1987
https://www.bbc.co.uk/programmes/b0078wbr

Stress Relief From Laughter?, 2023
www.mayoclinic.org/healthy-lifestyle/stress-management/in-depth/stress-relief/art-20044456

The Happiness Project, Body Worlds Museum, Amsterdam
www.bodyworlds.nl/en/

ibid.

Betty-Anne Heggie, 'The Healing Power of Laughter', *Journal of Hospital Medicine*, 2019 May; 14(5): 320.
www.ncbi.nlm.nih.gov/pmc/articles/PMC6609137/

Anti-happiness

The Happiness Project, Body Worlds Museum, Amsterdam
www.bodyworlds.nl/en/

Rick Hanson, *Resilient: 12 Tools for Transforming Everyday Happiness Into Lasting Happiness*, Rider, 2018

Spike Milligan, *Adolf Hitler: My Part in His Downfall*, Penguin, 2012

Viktor E. Frankl, *Man's Search for Meaning*, Rider, 2004

Dr Paul Yong
www.drpaulwong.com

Exploring habits and addictions

The Happiness Project, Body Worlds Museum, Amsterdam
www.bodyworlds.nl/en/

Katherine Arlinghaus & Craig Johnston, 'The Importance of Creating Habits and Routine', *Am J Lifestyle Med.* 2019 Mar-Apr; 13(2): 142–144.
https://www.ncbi.nlm.nih.gov/pmc/articles/PMC6378489/

James Clear, *Atomic Habits*, Random House Business, 2018

IB: Happiness Survey

We Are Family

Kerstin Uvnas-Moberg, Linda Handlin & Maria Petersson, 'Self-soothing behaviors with particular reference to oxytocin release induced by non-noxious sensory stimulation', *Front Psychol.* 2014; 5: 1529.
www.ncbi.nlm.nih.gov/pmc/articles/PMC4290532/

Relationships and Communities
www.mentalhealth.org.uk/explore-mental-health/statistics/relationships-community-statistics

Alison Huang, David L Roth, Tom Cidav, Shang-En Chung, Halima Amjad, Roland J Thorpe, Cynthia M Boyd & Thomas K Cudjoe, 'Social isolation and 9-year dementia risk in community-dwelling Medicare beneficiaries in the United States', *Journal of the American Geriatrics Society*, March 2023, Volume71, Issue 3, pp 765-773 https://agsjournals.onlinelibrary.wiley.com/doi/full/10.1111/jgs.18140

Robby Berman, *Social isolation, loneliness linked to increased risk of all-cause mortality*, (2023) www.medicalnewstoday.com/articles/social-isolation-loneliness-linked-to-increased-mortality-risk-research-finds

Patricia A Thomas, Hui Liu & Debra Umberson, 'Family Relationships and Well-Being', *Innov Aging.*, 2017 Nov, 1(3), igx025. https://www.ncbi.nlm.nih.gov/pmc/articles/PMC5954612/

Elena Delgado, Cristina Serna, Isabel Martinez & Edie Cruise, 'Parental Attachment and Peer Relationships in Adolescence: A Systematic Review', *Int J Environ Res Public Health.*, 2022 Jan 18;19(3) https://pubmed.ncbi.nlm.nih.gov/35162088/

Julianne Holt-Lunstad, Timothy B Smith, Mark Baker, Tyler Harris & David Stephenson, 'Loneliness and social isolation as risk factors for mortality: a meta-analytic review', *Perspect Psychol Sci.* 2015 Mar, 10(2): 227-37 https://pubmed.ncbi.nlm.nih.gov/25910392/

Love, Actually is...

Love Actually
Directed by Richard Curtis, Working Title Films

Guaranteed Joy With Richard Curtis podcast, Episode 73
https://simonsinek.com/podcast/episodes/guaranteed-joy-with-richard-curtis/

Marissa A Harrison & Jennifer C Shortall, 'Women and men in love: who really feels it and says it first?', *J Soc Psychol.* 2011 Nov-Dec;151(6):727-36.
https://pubmed.ncbi.nlm.nih.gov/22208110/

Hai-Jiang Li, Jian-Zhou Sun, Qing-Lin Zhang, Don-Tao Wei, Wen-Fu Li, Todd Jackson, Glenn Hitchman & Jiang Qiu, *Neuroanatomical* 'Differences between Men and Women in Help-Seeking Coping Strategy', *Sci Rep.* 2014 Jul 16;4:5700.
https://pubmed.ncbi.nlm.nih.gov/25027617/

Sari M van Anders, Jeffrey Steiger & , Katherine L Goldey, 'Effects of gendered behaviour on testosterone in women and men', *Proc Natl Acad Sci U S A.* 2015 Nov 10;112(45):13805-10.
https://pubmed.ncbi.nlm.nih.gov/26504229/

Differences Between Men and Women
https://relationship-institute.com/differences-between-men-and-women/

Why do pets have such a positive impact on our lives?

New Pet Ownership Challenges Emerging Post Pandemic, 2022
www.pdsa.org.uk/press-office/latest-news/paw-report-reveals-new-pet-ownership-challenges-emerging-post-pandemic

The Power of Pets, (2018)
https://newsinhealth.nih.gov/2018/02/power-pets

www.pawsinwork.com

Ann Robinson, 'Dogs have a magic effect', *The Guardian* (2020)
www.theguardian.com/society/2020/mar/17/dogs-have-a-magic-effect-the-power-of-pets-on-our-mental-health

Our Chosen Hobbies

Dr Jaime L Kurtz, *Six Reasons to Get a Hobby* (2015)
www.psychologytoday.com/gb/blog/happy-trails/201509/six-reasons-get-hobby

Music for the soul

The Happiness Project, Body Worlds Museum, Amsterdam
www.bodyworlds.nl/en/

Dr Elizabeth Scott, *How Music Can Be Therapeutic* (2020)
www.verywellmind.com/how-and-why-music-therapy-is-effective-3145190

ibid.

Everybody's Free (to wear sunscreen), Something for Everybody album, (1998) Baz Lurhmann, (featuring Quindon Tarver), based on an essay Wear Sunscreen by Mary Schmich in The Chicago Tribune, June 1997

Set You Free, Electronic Pleasure album, 1995, N-Trance, featuring Kelly Llorenna, written by N-Trance

Everywhere, Tango in the Night album, 1987, Fleetwood Mac, written by Christine McVie

Material Girl

The Happiness Project, Body Worlds Museum, Amsterdam
www.bodyworlds.nl/en/

Sheena S Iyengar & Mark R Lepper, 'When choice is demotivating: Can one desire too much of a good thing?' *Journal of Personality and Social Psychology*, 2020, 79(6), 995–1006.
https://psycnet.apa.org/doiLanding?doi=10.1037%2F0022-351
4.79.6.995

Ramsey's Kitchen Nightmares, TV show
Channel 4 Television Corporation

Angus Deaton & Daniel Kahneman, 'High income improves evaluation of life but not emotional well-being', *Proceedings of the National Academy of Sciences*, Vol. 107 | No. 38
www.pnas.org/doi/full/10.1073/pnas.1011492107

Arwa Mahdawi, 'The biggest lie the rich ever told? That money can't buy you happiness', *The Guardian* (Mar 2023)
https://www.theguardian.com/commentisfree/2023/mar/14/the-biggest-lie-the-rich-ever-told-that-money-cant-buy-you-happiness

Timothy Ferris, *The 4-Hour Work Week*, Vermillion, 2011

Vicki Robin and Joe Dominguez, *Your Money or Your Life*, Penguin Publishing Group, 2008

Booked it. Packed it. F* *cked off...

"Booked it. Packed it. F* *cked off..." Peter Kay, Live At The Top Of The Tower, 2000

Caroline Castrillon, *Why Taking Vacation Time Can Save Your Life* (2021) www.forbes.com/sites/carolinecastrillon/2021/05/23/why-taking-vacation-time-could-save-your-life/?sh=f8ef0524de0b

Long working hours increasing deaths from heart disease and stroke: WHO, ILO (2021)
www.who.int/news/item/17-05-2021-long-working-hours-increasing-deaths-from-heart-disease-and-stroke-who-ilo

Rebecca Zucker, *How Taking a Vacation Improves Your Well-Being* (2023)
https://hbr.org/2023/07/how-taking-a-vacation-improves-your-well-being

ibid.

A Bit of Alone Time

A.A. Milne, *Pooh's Little Instruction Book*, Methuen Winnie the Pooh, 1996

Thomas Oppong, *Time Alone is a Tool For Self Awareness*, 2023
https://medium.com/mind-cafe/solitude-time-alone-is-a-tool-for-self-awareness-43f8e9163950

How to Practise Self-Awareness Podcast 178, Stephen Warley
https://lifeskillsthatmatter.com/podcast/how-to-practice-self-awareness/

Amy Morin, *7 Science-Backed Reasons You Should Spend More Time Alone*, (2017)
www.forbes.com/sites/amymorin/2017/08/05/7-science-backed-reasons-you-should-spend-more-time-alone/?sh=2793e99d1b7e

David Kundtz, *The One You Feed* podcast, *The Art of Stopping* by (April 2021)
www.oneyoufeed.net/the-art-of-stopping/

Sleepy Bunnies

Twinkle, Twinkle Little Star, written by Jane Taylor in Rhymes for the Nursery (1806)

Arianna Huffington, *The Sleep Revolution*, Harmony, 2016

Shawn Stevenson, *Sleep Smarter*, Hay House UK, 2016

Good Sleep for Good Health, April 21
https://newsinhealth.nih.gov/2021/04/good-sleep-good-health

T Roehrs, T Roth, 'Sleep, sleepiness, and alcohol use', *Alcohol Res Health*. 2001, 25(2):101-9. PMID: 11584549; PMCID: PMC6707127.

https://pubmed.ncbi.nlm.nih.gov/11584549/

Basal Body Temperature (BBT) Charting

https://www.peacehealth.org/medical-topics/id/hw202058

What Happens to Your Body When You Sleep, 2021
www.webmd.com/sleep-disorders/what-happens-body-during-sleep

This Works sleep spray
www.thisworks.com/products/deep-sleep-pillow-spray-75ml

1C Happiness and work

It's all work, work, work...

Walt Disney's *Snow White and the Seven Dwarfs*, directed by David Hand, 1937

One-Third of Your Life is Spent at Work
www.gettysburg.edu/news/stories?id=79db7b34-630c-4f49-ad32-4ab9ea48e72b

More Than Three-Quarters of the UK Not Happy at Work, blog post, 2023
www.openstudycollege.com/blog/more-than-three-quarters-of-the-uk-not-happy-at-work?queryID=266722a1519108919c6f85 1e63c3b758&objectID=102961-0

Benjamin Todd, *We reviewed over 60 studies about what makes for a dream job. Here's what we found.* (2014 – updated 2023)
https://80000hours.org/career-guide/job-satisfaction/

Julian Bazley
www.fitterlonger.com

Dale Carnegie, *How to Enjoy Your Life and Your Job*, General Press, 2018

James Thomas
www.dogsofhenley.com

Understanding Your Personality Profile

https://actioncoach.co.uk/free-disc-profile

https://www.thomas.co

https://www.insights.com

Mark Van Rol
markvanrol.actioncoach.co.uk

Let's be SMART about this

Viktor E. Frankl, *Man's Search for Meaning*, Rider, 2004

Kimberlee Leonard & Rob Watts, *The Ultimate Guide to S.M.A.R.T. Goals*, 2022
www.forbes.com/advisor/business/smart-goals/

Lady Luck or hard graft?

Gary Player quote
www.calmpeople.co.uk/the-harder-i-practise-the-luckier-i-get/

World Happiness Report 2023, Sustainable Development Solutions Network
https://worldhappiness.report/ed/2023/world-happiness-trust-and-social-connections-in-times-of-crisis/

Daniel Kahneman, *Thinking Fast and Slow*, Penguin, 2012

1D Happiness over time

Happiness over time

The Happiness Project, Body Worlds Museum, Amsterdam
www.bodyworlds.nl/en/

Matt Weiking, CEO, The Happiness Research Institute
www.happinessresearchinstitute.com/_files/ugd/928487_86c
12c375d3a468c89efedd3cbf56bb8.pdf

Parenthood

The Happiness Project, Body Worlds Museum, Amsterdam
www.bodyworlds.nl/en/

Viewing Life Like a Child

Lara B Aknin, J Kiley Hamlin & Elizabeth W Dunn, 'Giving Leads
to Happiness in Young Children', *PLoS ONE*, 2012, 7(6): e39211
https://journals.plos.org/plosone/article?id=10.1371/journal.
pone.0039211

Section 2: MOVE

The Happiness Project, Body Worlds Museum, Amsterdam
www.bodyworlds.nl/en/

Jenny J Roe, Catherine Ward Thompson, Peter A Aspinall, Mark J
Brewer, Elizabeth I Duff, David Miller, Richard Mitchell & Angela
Clow, 'Green Space and Stress: Evidence From Cortisol Measures
in Deprived Urban Communities', *Int J Environ Res Public Health.*
2013 Sep 2;10(9):4086-103.
https://www.ncbi.nlm.nih.gov/pmc/articles/PMC3799530/

Nature and Mental Health
www.mind.org.uk/information-support/tips-for-everyday-living/
nature-and-mental-health/how-nature-benefits-mental-health/

Elaine M Murtagh, Marie H Murphy & Janne Boone-Heinonen, 'Walking – the first steps in cardiovascular disease prevention', *Curr Opin Cardiol.* 2010 Sep;25(5):490-6.
www.ncbi.nlm.nih.gov/pmc/articles/PMC3098122/

MyFitnessPal
www.myfitnesspal.com

Nutracheck Calorie Counter
www.nutracheck.co.uk/CaloriesIn/#url

Section 3: EAT

UK/NHS Live Well Eatwell Guide:
www.nhs.uk/live-well/eat-well/food-guidelines-and-food-labels/the-eatwell-guide/

Madonna Mamerow, Joni Mettler, Kirk English, Shanon Casperson, Emily Arentson-Lantz, Melinda Sheffield-Moore, Donald Layman, & Douglas Paddon-Jones, 'Dietary Protein Distribution Positively Influences 24-h Muscle Protein Synthesis in Healthy Adults', *The Journal of Nutrition*, 2014,144(6), 876–880
https://doi.org/10.3945/jn.113.185280

Drinkaware
www.drinkaware.co.uk

Live Happy
www.livehappy.app

Food Standards Agency
www.food.gov.uk

British Nutrition Foundation
www.nutrition.org.uk

Mental Health Foundation
www.mentalhealth.org.uk

EPILOGUE:

Delphin Be Grand Hotel
www.delphinhotel.com/en/delphin-be-grand-resort

ACKNOWLEDGEMENTS

I would like to thank the following people for their contributions, support, and professional knowledge. Without them, writing this book would have been a lot harder and nowhere near as useful to you, dear reader!

Firstly, my family support network: My husband, Sam, for putting up with me having to squirrel myself away many times to write and be creative. My parents, for listening to me harp on about this book for many months. My sister, Caroline, for also listening to me harp on but being my sounding board on many of the topics, to ensure I wasn't going off the rails too much. My cousin, Hannah, for reading the very first draft of this book whilst on a train to Amsterdam with me on a girls' weekend away, and for making very positive noises throughout the whole journey!

Secondly, my wonderful and loyal clients, and my Live Happy colleagues – they have given me most of my inspiration for this book and many real-life examples.

Thirdly, my publishing team – they have helped me to craft this book into something that I am so proud to publish and be in the public domain, and kept me enjoying the book writing process from start to finish.

ABOUT THE AUTHOR

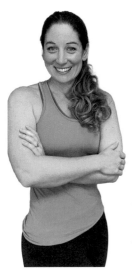

Rebecca Myers is the founder of Live Happy – the health and well-being company. It consists of a network of physical gym facilities, a holistic app product, and a host of corporate health and well-being consultative services.

Her qualifications span from personal trainer, nutrition coach, mental health first aider, counsellor, BSc business graduate, mum to two beautiful but demanding 'tweenage' boys, and wife to long-suffering husband, Sam – who has put up with hours of looking after the children whilst this book has been written, plus being IT support to ensure all the words aren't lost!

www.livehappy.group

www.linkedin.com/in/rebeccamyers2

www.instagram.com/work_in_your_work_out

www.facebook.com/wiywo